Outsmart Your Addiction

Jason Giles M.D.

ACKNOWLEDGMENTS

It is impossible for me to thank all the people who made this book possible. First off, I'd like to thank God for all the help and grace to make something worthwhile of my life. Right after that comes my wife, Rebecca, and our children Truman and Ava. If I have striven to be a better husband and father it's because these three deserve the best I can be.
There is nothing to compare with the feeling of having a true ride-or-die partner in life. Dr./Mrs. Giles is as good as they come. Thanks for encouraging me to write this book and thanks for all the years my love.

Next are my parents. My own father passed away in 2014, but the impression he left on me is deep. I was afraid of him, I wanted to be like him, and to be not at all like him. In the end, we just accepted each other. My mother did her best to make life at home bearable during my dad's struggles with alcohol. Often I was angry with her for not making everything perfect, but that is the immature wish of a child. My mother taught me perseverance and humility. She is a good mom. Also on the parent list of thanks is my father-in-law Eldred. Whenever I have an ethical quandary, I simply imagine what Papa would do and the way forward becomes clear.

My two oldest friends, Mark and David, are my brothers. They've been around since middle school and we'll be there for each other until the end. I love both you guys and wouldn't be here without you. My friends in the new millennium are fast-tracking to brotherhood too: John, Victor, Kenny, and David D. They give me the gift of candor. They're honest about their lives, and they patiently listen to me when I'm knotted up over a problem.

I can't let this page go by without thanking my friends, mentors, sponsors and sponsees in Alcoholics Anonymous. I am not a representative or spokesman for A.A., but they as much as anyone gave me guidance and support when I needed it most.

And extra special thanks to Francine for spitting in my soup.

Now look, making a list like this is impossible. I'm flooded with memories and emotions thinking about all the people who made this book come to be. In the spirit of covert recognition for the part you played, and you know who you are, THANK YOU!

This work is dedicated to my patients.

CONTENTS

CONTENTS (Con't)

-1-
I PROMISED MYSELF I'D NEVER USE AGAIN

The operating room thermometer reads a chilly fifty-five Fahrenheit, but I can't stop sweating. It's been more than twelve hours since I last injected fentanyl into the battered vein at the crease of my left elbow. Despite the frigid air, my surgical gown sticks to the thin cotton/poly blend of my soaked scrub pajamas. I am in my third year of training to be an anesthesiologist. I spent my first year on the other side of the drape in surgery. I have "M.D." after my name, which sounds significant, but in this room, everyone outranks me. I'm dehydrated from sweating, and from deliberately not drinking anything in anticipation of the long case ahead. Trust me, you don't want to have to pee when they clamp the aorta.

This is the most difficult case I've ever done, and maybe the most difficult operation in medicine, even more than neurosurgery or a heart transplantation. Our patient has a lengthening tear in his aorta – the largest artery in the body. The surgeons are planning to replace the patient's entire ascending aorta and arch, the branches of the "Amazon River of Life," that feed fresh blood to the heart and brain. We must operate now or he will be dead by sundown. I'm worried for him, but I'm more worried for me. If it all goes sideways, I fear I'll be kicked out of the operating room, my residency, the hospital, and probably medicine altogether.

I am the junior member of an elite team of doctors, nurses, and perfusionists who are about to kill a man to save his life. The candy-cane-shaped aortic arch has off-ramps to the heart, head, and arms. They have to be clamped during the replacement with the new arch. The prosthetic blood vessel is made of Dacron, the same fiber used to make shag carpeting and most of the material in my clingy scrubs. Heart surgeons routinely go around the beating heart with a bypass pump, but we can't use it here or the patient will back-bleed to death from the arteries in his neck. We must stop the circulation completely for most of an hour.

Our patient is an especially tall forty-year-old man. He has Marfan syndrome, a disease of collagen weakness. Almost all the body's structural integrity depends on the cross-linked strength of this humble protein. In Marfan, the structural weakness results in weak arteries and lax ligaments. His fingers are so flexible that his fingertips point backwards at right angles when he holds the pen to sign the consent form for surgery.

He's had the ticking time bomb of his flimsy aorta, shredding itself with each beat of his heart, for the past year. Abraham Lincoln may have had Marfan syndrome, his height and spider-like fingers offering clues. Professional basketball player Isaiah Austin has Marfan syndrome. When our patient felt a ripping pain in the center of his chest, he called 911 and passed out. He arrives this morning to the pre-op holding area, his blood pressure kept artificially low to slow progression of the aortic tear. He smells of the antibiotic a nurse used to scrub his washboard chest.

The surgeons have their own informed consent forms spelling out the possible risks from the surgery itself: heart attack, stroke, blindness, and so forth. Anesthesia paperwork is my job, and I explain the risks to this man. Once his BP is lowered and stabilized, his pain goes away. He is unnaturally calm as I go over the things that could go wrong. Stroke, death, infection, allergic reaction, kidney failure, bladder injury, nerve damage, blindness, seizures, vocal cord damage from the breathing tube. I make sure he understands what he might be getting into. As he signs, I add, "I almost forgot, chipped teeth."

"How are you going to chip my teeth?"

"When we put the tube in. The laryngoscope can sometimes wedge against the teeth." Our patient has the lantern jaw of the sixteenth president. "Don't worry about that, though. I'll be extra careful."

He looks at me for an uncomfortable extra moment as we both envision what I just told him. He trusts me not to chip his teeth. More important, he trusts me to look out for him while he's asleep. He smiles and his shoulders relax. Years from now I will realize that the best part of being an anesthesiologist is when the patient invests his trust in me. Don't misunderstand, the physiology and the struggle in the OR are sublime, but the human connection when a patient says, "I trust you" is without equal. I want to be worthy of this confidence, but today I don't feel worthy.

A few hours earlier I made a solemn promise to whatever is out there that I would never use again. The drug I swore off, fentanyl, has a short half-life and I was already in early-stage withdrawal. This morning I looked in the mirror, and for the hundredth consecutive day, I vowed to put it behind me. I was just about to give in to the overwhelming psychological and physiological pressure when I got the call that we had an emergency arch. Maybe we can make it through together. I'll stay clean so I can help him, and helping him will keep me clean.

There is a lot to set up for these cases, and I was put right to work in OR 17. Infusions, pressure-measuring transducers, motorized operating table, split endotracheal tubes, and enough crushed ice for a lavish seafood buffet are all arranged. The blood bank is alerted, and we need special antibiotics that work at a cold temperature. Arch replacement is the surgical equivalent of getting an astronaut on the moon. All the preparations give me another focus instead of myself.

Like everyone who's ever become hooked, I didn't plan to be. I just wanted a little break in the routine. I had been through drinking to the point of pancreatitis. White-hot upper abdominal pain boring through to my spine helped me shy away from alcohol. Marijuana left a sticky film over my thoughts. I could hardly concentrate the day after smoking it. Pot was out. My free-floating anxiety is of the sort that a little something makes a big difference in my ability to handle life. Just knowing I could take something up around the bend was a comfort. Kind of like how it is easy not to smoke on a plane when you know you can't and when you have a few smokes in your pocket.

My brief relief was now back to collect the bill. I began with the naïve idea that I could control and enjoy my intravenous drug use. Controlling it turned out to be not so enjoyable, and in a series of personal "bests," my tolerance had trampled past unmanageability and into chemical enslavement. In some form, the drug infringes upon every thought.

For weeks now I wake up sick. This isn't a touch of the flu or the cramps after eating bad fish. I'm malaria sick. Dengue fever sick. My mattress has a moldy funk from the nightly sweat soaking that never has a chance to dry. The instant my eyes are open I must run to the toilet to avoid disaster on the mattress. My head feels like Anton Chigurh bolted it a few times. I shower in the dark and try to thaw my frozen marrow under the hot water. I tell myself every morning I'm almost halfway out. Twenty-four hours from now and the worst will be behind me.

My car drives itself to the hospital. I look up to the black sky beyond the illuminated helipad and tell god to go fuck himself. The automatic doors hiss open. I walk past the security guard. His powder blue shirt is pilled and faded. He glances up from his newspaper, barely recognizing another in the parade of young doctors filing in to the UC Davis Medical Center.

Once I am inside it is even harder to keep my promise. The fentanyl is only one floor above me. Nobody suspects that I'm stealing narcotics and shooting them in the bathroom after work. They couldn't. I've been much too clever. Lately I haven't been so good at hiding my tracks. I want to run back to the security guard, Frank, and say, "Hey, so you know, it's me. All that missing dope? Yeah, guilty. I need help and I don't want to die." Instead I walk in just like any other day at the office, only my office is a Level I trauma hospital.

The death part, the think I want to blurt out to Frank – well, today that doesn't sound so bad to me. I am in an internal war between keeping quiet and screaming for help. Fear has an unbroken streak longer than Dimaggio's. I bargain with these inner voices to keep my secret for one more day, but only on the solemn promise that if I can't keep the needle out of my arm for twenty-four hours then I will ask for help. Tomorrow. I keep shooting up…one day at a time.

In this corner of the hospital I am a rising star, the golden boy of the anesthesia department and probably headed for a life in academic medicine. If you looked closely over the past six months, I'm looking literally a little golden too. Not yet jaundiced but clearly a shade of pale yellow. Sallow you could say and you'd not be wrong. The sleep deprivation, vampire schedule, and poor diet have not helped my look.

I always have on a long sateen Gore-Tex gown from the OR surgical supply. I wear it backwards, that is normal-facing, with the opening in the front over my scrubs. My arms are splattered with bruises and needle-marks, but you can't see them under long sleeves. Back in the beginning I just shot up in the distal cephalic vein, right underneath the sweep of my watchband. Now that tributary is a hard rope. I can't even wear a watch.

It is stupid to inject in your feet (hydrostatic pressure), so I never do that. I cadge 32-gauge needles from the ophthalmology department to minimize vein trauma, but nobody's perfect after hundreds of injections. Sometimes I miss and inject alongside the vein. Sometimes I go right through both walls. The law of averages. I'm not going to do this forever anyway. It's a phase, and today I'm finished with it. Twenty-three and a half hours to go.

I was supposed to be doing anesthesia for endoscopies down in the CT scanner. I was on trauma call yesterday, and the scheduler will try to give the post-call guy an easy day. I hate it, though, spending the day underground with the endoscopists. Stale jokes (read the card!) and the patients are sick. You are far away from help if something bad happens. Instead I stand inside the surgery department entrance looking at the massive whiteboard with the day's cases neatly written. I'm trying to force down a buttermilk donut and cup of oversweet Constant Comment when Dr. Hanowell nonchalantly asks me if I want to do a total arch.

"An arch?" I stammer.

"Yep," he pulls the lever on the coffee tank.

"Circ arrest?" I ask.

"See you in room 17," he says as he whistles off in that direction.

☐

-2-
DOES EVERYONE KNOW?

The department chairman, Peter Moore, is running the board this morning. He smiles at me. Peter went to a selective science school as a boy, but he has the rugged handsomeness of a rugby player. His Newcastle accent is thick.

"I still remember me first aaach," he says. He tells the board nurse to get one of the CRNAs to do the GI cases and writes HANOWELL/GILES in the anesthesia column with a blue, squeaky, dry-erase marker.

Enthusiastically, he adds, "Remember, when they fiddle-fart around with the carotids, look out!"

Arch cases are rare, especially semi-elective ones like this. I'd already been on an acute trauma broken arch when I was a first-year medical student. It was the first time I'd held a living human heart. The pretty young blonde had been on a motorcycle when it crashed. The driver, her boyfriend, was getting all the attention because he was unconscious in the other trauma bay. She was talking as she rolled in on a gurney. She sat up, looked at us with pale blue frightened eyes, tried to speak, and fell back dead. The surgeon splashed antiseptic on her bare chest and cut through to her breastbone with a single slash. We spread her chest with a Finochietto, twirling the handle to reveal a twitching heart in fibrillation. Dr. Blaisdell, the surgery chairman, showed me how to manually pump her heart with my two cupped hands. "Like a crocodile!" he said. I felt her heart go limp and she never awoke.

Aortic disruption repair, with any warning to the hospital team, is uncommon. There's an awful joke about the twenty-year reunion of all the ruptured aortic arch survivors getting together…*both of them.* For the surgeons doing the case, the most junior among them had already completed a five-year surgery residency. The nurses and perfusionists were all senior pros. My supervising staff, Dr. Hanowell, was a cardiac-trained professor who split time between the UC Davis and Stanford hospitals. Lee would have been at home in a wartime British hospital. He wore a triangular moustache, and his smooth features echoed an ancient marble bust, pale and worn down by the centuries. His eyes flashed whenever he was discussing a point of anesthesia-craft.

I was excited to be asked to serve on this case. The norepenipherine pulsing into my bloodstream by my adrenal glands raised in me an anxious hyper-focus. I told myself I was happy to be going through the torture of withdrawal this morning because, of all days, today I needed to be sharp. Arch cases take a long time, too. By the time we finish, I will be nearly through the worst part of the case and will need just a bit of willpower to push across the finish line to get my IV drug phase behind me. Nobody will ever know.

The greatest advance in the history of surgery is anesthesia. Without an anesthetic, surgical prowess was judged in the pre-anesthesia era by how fast a doctor could saw through bone. The other magical achievement in surgery is infection control. Mostly that is done by avoiding contamination in the first place – sterile instruments, alcohol to clean the skin, and with the preemptive use of antibiotics. Temperature plays a major role in reducing post-op infection. It took us a while to figure this out, but warm surgical patients fight infection much better than cold ones. Normal body temperature is 37° Celsius. Mr. Marfan is going down to 18° Celsius, or about 64° Fahrenheit. His head will be packed in crushed ice. We are aiming for a nasal probe temperature of 14°C, or 57°F.

At 18°C, cells metabolize at a tiny fraction of their usual pace. The brain and heart are good for about five minutes – max – without blood flow at normal body temperature. Cold buys time – at least an hour, maybe longer. The drawback is that cold wreaks hell on systems we want to run normally, like white blood cells to fight infection and enzymes that cause blood to clot. It is a Faustian bargain to refrigerate a person to save him. We literally kill him – he will have no brain activity – for about an hour.

Anesthetic management is hard at these temperatures, too. Mr. Marfan will require a bucket of pain medicine and gas to tolerate the scalpels and bone saws that are about to open his chest. A spike in blood pressure from felt pain could cause his frangible arch to split in twain. Too much anesthesia and his pressure will plummet, and his heart will starve for oxygen right before the toughest job of its life. We have the luxury of a long post-op recovery time, not needing to wake him up right after the case. Dr. Hanowell and I agree to employ high-dose opiates during and especially at the end of the case. They provide a smooth, deep background of pain and consciousness suppression. He will be on a ventilator for a few days anyway. I sign out 200 cc of fentanyl from the OR pharmacy, roughly twice as much as our patient will need.

If we nail the titration of gas and I.V. anesthetic, the surgeons can get the bypass cannulas up the femoral vessels in his thighs to a point below the tear in his aorta, all without splitting the weakened aorta. As the patient's blood is removed, cooled, and returned by the perfusionists, I will pack the patient's head in ice. All this cold makes anesthetic management tough. The body basically stops metabolizing the drugs, and they would hang around indefinitely except for the constant blood loss. It is common to replace nearly all of a person's blood during this kind of a case. We try our best to recapture blood lost with a special machine that rinses it and saves the red cells, but it is an uphill battle. The blood bank phone rings off the hook during the case.

Before we go back to the OR, I get some Imodium out of my backpack. One of the more unpleasant features of opiate withdrawal is the loosening of the bowels. The last thing I need today is that kind of an accident in the OR. I wash the capsules down with the last of the cold tea. I put on a second scrub top in the locker room: an extra layer for warmth. Peter offers more chipper Aussie encouragement.

I go down the hall to the surgical ICU and transfer all the pumps and monitors to the poles on Mr. M's hospital bed. He tells me about how he met his wife when he was camping down in Yosemite Valley, slurring through the tale as the sedative I give him takes effect. We get to the meat locker that is our OR and he comments on the arctic temperature. I carefully transfer the pumps and monitors off his bed over to ours at the head of the table, and we slide him over. At well over six feet tall he needs a table extension to support his overhang. Induction of anesthesia goes smoothly, and after only forty-five minutes, all our infusion and monitoring catheters are in. No pressure spikes or crashes, first hurdle crossed.

The surgeons put in their big pipes, and the chest is opened with a nitrogen-powered reciprocating saw in a smooth pass. We continue to cool him until the heart slows, and then just stops. We keep cooling by running the pumped blood in tubes through an ice bath. Coagulation goes to hell, he leaks from every cut tissue edge, and the blood bank brings another twenty pints of blood. There isn't much for us to do up top except shift from foot to foot to stay warm. No heartbeat, lungs off, urine output zero. His pH is 7.2, not too bad for a dead man. The whole room is transfixed stitch by stitch. The head surgeon, Dr. Delius, wears a small video camera attached to a headband on his brow; the ten of us in the room watch his nimble needlework. I'm grateful for the two-hour distraction and the cold. I'm hardly sweating.

We get by on hypothermia as an anesthetic until the repair is complete. With no brain function, there is no pain. I confirm a quiet mind with a special surface EEG, though the ice keeps soaking off the adhesive on Mr. Marfan's forehead. The aortic repair is blood-tight and Delius releases the. The blood is warmed slowly via the bypass machine. I remove the cranial ice bags. Coagulation is for shit, and he leaks worse than ever. We wait to fix it because most of the poor clotting is due to the cold. We are so busy that I've forgotten all about my own discomfort. All that hiking pays off and his heart leaps to life. Warmer and warmer the EEG starts to come off a flat line brainwave. I add a little anesthetic. The room nurse switches on the heat in the OR and my sweating returns.

We begin working in fentanyl as he gets warmer. I figure most of it is still being sucked away from the operating field and estimate generously the replacement of the narcotic. His pressure on the arteriogram tracing is a red line wiggling across the black monitor. It spikes, then it plummets as they manipulate his carotid arteries, just like Peter warned. I "tap the brakes" with a squirt of beta-blocker and goose the pressure with a little nor-epi(nephrine). I try to anticipate the changes, dancing with the surgeons and perfusionists. We work together flawlessly.

I add clotting factors to his main IV and soon we see small clots forming in the operative field. A chest drainage tube is placed for later monitoring and we "come off" bypass. His heart is carrying its own workload and looks good. Snappy. The ventilator fills and empties his pink lungs. His EEG shows he's still deeply under but with a brain that roughly works – a hopeful indication. The Dacron graft in place of his old rotten aorta quivers and thrums with each heartbeat.

The surgeons close the delicate pericardium and then wire the breastbone shut. The skin is clipped closed. I put the several new pumps and monitor boxes back on the hospital bed. We "1-2-3" him back to the ICU bed and wheel Mr. M back to room 2 in the cardiac surgical ICU, or SI-2.

I give a report to the SI nurse, Doug, nicknamed The Wookie, because of his bushy mop of hair and his seamless flow of beard. The red squiggle appears on the ICU monitor as three nurses move the pumps, tubes, and drains where they are supposed to go.

"Are you okay?" asks the Wookie.

"Yeah, just a bit fried after this case."

He keeps his eyes on me until it starts to feel weird. He eventually releases me. Does everyone know? Mr. M is stable-ish and my Imodium has worn off.

I go to the call room to take a shower; the hot water loosens the knotted muscles in my neck. The rest of the fentanyl is in my backpack, calling me. I look in the foggy mirror at my skinny reflection, arms covered in bruises. I probably weigh about one hundred sixty pounds. This does not look healthy on a six-two frame. The heat and the glimpse of myself combine to bolster my resolve not to use. I put on clean scrubs. A fresh gown covers my arms. I get out of that call room and away from my backpack to check on the patient.

The case from start to finish has taken ten hours. The afternoon sun yellows the rice fields west of Sacramento. I go back to SI-2 and complete the anesthetic paperwork. Here I must get through another narrow gate: the record. So far, I have recorded the actual amount of fentanyl Mr. M received during the case. This number is somewhere around five milligrams of the potent narcotic (about eighty times stronger than morphine), a good amount for this case, but I have checked out ten milligrams from the pharmacy. If I write in a few more doses on the record, I can take one or more of the remaining vials. They are twenty milliliter ampules, super-sized fentanyl, instead of the usual 5 ml ones. The patient is comfortable and I am uncomfortable. If I fudge the record, then the pharmacy won't have a discrepancy. If I leave it accurate as it is now, then I am at least twelve more hours away from my next opportunity to score the drug.

I dither with the nurses and surgeons who shuttle between their posts and the ICU to check on the total arch. The take-back rate is high for this kind of operation, and we all want to give him at least a few hours before we leave. The best team to fix any problems is the team that caused them, should they arise. The bleeding into the chest drainage tubes slows and the urine output picks up, both good signs.

It is safe to eat dinner since the patient is more stable by the hour. I go to the basement cafeteria and prowl the steam tables. I get a plate of something and a bucket of diet coke. My bowels are a troupe of acrobats. I sip another Imodium. I'm seated at the long green melamine tables, and I look over my cases for the next day.

They are routine ortho foot cases. I make calls to tomorrow's patients from the staff phone by the banquette. I make clumsy stabs at the buttons and more than a few tries before getting the number right. I don't like getting them on the phone, but I like talking with them. Of course, they are anxious for the big (bunion) surgery tomorrow. I spend a few minutes confirming their medical history and reason for the operation. The chat is mostly social with an aim toward reassurance. They feel better because they know their anesthesiologist cares. They will take or skip the right medications, which will in turn make my job easier tomorrow.

If I'm even here tomorrow.

-3-
I SHOOT THE WHOLE THING

One of the major problems with drug addiction is the mental space it occupies. You're always mega-hyper-multitasking. One would think that life and training to be an anesthesiologist would be challenging enough. Adding the spice of a rapacious drug dependency on a short-acting narcotic makes everything complex and challenging. Doing cases with essentially no narcotics, such as ear tubes or CT scans, means you are in a jam. Weekend off? Most residents consider that Shangri-La. Have a fentanyl habit to support? You're fucked. Fortunately, I only get a whole weekend off every other month. Failing to pace out the narcotics leaves me open to suffering, and the desiccated gnawing of withdrawal.

But today is different. Look what I have accomplished already! It has been almost twenty-four hours since I last shot up, and despite soaking my scrubs with sweat every hour, I might make it this time. Really, only another day to go. I've never done it, but I could call in sick. Wouldn't be a lie, just can't say why I am sick. Two days off this painkiller, and my will would be like iron. I'd be done with drugs and someday it would make a great story — a story that I would be buried with me.

Enough time has passed with Mr. M recovering in his intensive care bed for me to start thinking about going home for the day. I stop by again and look at his fluid balance and lung compliance. It is way too early to know if his brain will be okay. He has a long way to go still. Why can't I be sedated and ventilated for the next two days? I can't do that solo. I speak with Mrs. M and reassure her that everything went well in the case. We did a fine job and he is a fighter, I tell her. I'm trying to boost my own resolve and sip off his hopeful prognosis.

As a contingency, I have set aside two hundred fifty micrograms of fentanyl in a five-milliliter syringe. This amount was to be given to Mr. M at the start of the case, but the nursing staff already medicated him just before I picked him up in the ICU. I recorded it as a pre-op med and it is on the sheet. In the world of record keeping it has already been given to the patient. I could waste it in the trash or down the sink. In this case, it is such a small amount that its absence would raise no flags. Having made a fresh commitment to myself not to shoot any more fentanyl, I feel as though my chance is at hand to break free once and for all. Also, I'm riding high on the early success of the big case and feel like celebrating a little.

In the staff bathroom between the OR and the ICU, I snick the deadbolt and take a breath. I have with me everything I need to shoot the fentanyl, but I must be strong. The sink whispers softly for me to squirt the drug down the drain, but my aching marrow overrules the sink. I compromise and squirt the drug in my mouth. As a point of information, oral fentanyl is only about 50 percent absorbed as compared to injectable. A little edge off, and a micro celebration along with keeping my promise to myself not to shoot up. I've figured it out. At one-half bioavailability (compared to I.V.) I wasted half. Not bad. Every little thing gonna be alright.

The swig of fentanyl has no discernible effect on my withdrawal symptoms. Last month that amount, even orally, would have given me a velvet buzz. Two weeks ago, the same dose would have banished all the sick. Now it is a single, limp sandbag against a flood of suffering. I might as well have sipped a teaspoon of Constant Comment tea for the same amount of relief. This isn't a red flag; it's a parachute that failed to open. I am in way over my head, but I still think this is just a puzzle to be solved.

I leave the bathroom and head toward the second-floor pharmacy around the corner from the ICU, where I turn in my drug kit. I submit all the pink sheets and the unused drugs checked out this morning. They are put in a Ziploc bag for auditing by the pharmacist later. One might think, "I'll take out drugs from the vials and put back water or saline." Forget it. They check the density of the solutions returned with a refractometer. Any discrepancy triggers an analysis of what you claimed was morphine, fentanyl, or what have you. They will catch your lie.

I hand the bag to the pharmacy assistant and he signs off on the form that he received it. Back in the ICU, one last peek in at the patient: stable. I shoulder my backpack and make for the exit. Gold rays filter through low mottled clouds along the swollen Sacramento River. I drive toward the shafts of light feeling sick. I cross the causeway on Interstate 80.

The river is always swollen this time of year, and the Fremont Weir has filled the Yolo bypass with cold Sacramento River water. Instead of going home to my little two-bedroom house on Cowell Boulevard in Davis, I pull off an exit before at Levee Road. The motor of my oxidized white Acura sedan ticks as it cools in the evening air. I click the seat back two stops, open the sunroof, light a cigarette, and deeply breathe in the smoke.

I open the pencil case zipper pouch on my blue Cordura backpack to reveal two 20 ml vials of fentanyl citrate from Astra Zeneca. The red glow of my cigarette coal glints off the thin borosilicate glass. Momentarily, I consider throwing them both out the sunroof and into the swift water below. This thought is dispatched with the twisting of my guts and the squeezing in my vertebrae brought on by my plummeting serum narcotic level. I don't stand a chance out here all alone.

I snap open a clean syringe and easily draw up the thin clear liquid through a large bore needle, deftly unscrewing and swapping this one for a tiny 32-gauge micro fine needle. The process is automatic now. I don't use a tourniquet because I know where all my veins are by feel. I wipe an alcohol swab across my angry forearm and feel the tiny give of skin, then vein, two physical layers of resistance giving way. The needle tip finds its target: a show of dark blood at the hub. Still not too late to cancel the operation here. Just don't push the plunger. Shh.

Though low in viscosity, twenty milliliters of fentanyl can take a full minute to pass through such a fine needle. Thin needles make small holes, and there is less of a chance for back-bleeding, bruising, and infection. I already feel better even though I haven't depressed the thick sintered circle crowning the plunger's flange. I'm in control of how I will feel in the next minute. The chatter inside my head stops. I lean forward in quiet anticipation. I've never done this much fentanyl before, and the promise of relief coupled with the possibility of overdose is better than the drug itself. I don't want to die, but I can't go on much longer like this. I have a spiritual lightness at this moment of balanced control and abandon.

I decide to use only ten. Half the syringe and save the rest for later, or maybe even throw it away if I have the courage.

Who am I kidding?

I shoot the whole thing.

This isn't easy, mind you, keeping all those pounds-per-square-inch of pressure on a big syringe hubbed to a tiny needle in a fragile vein. As the drug starts to work its ligand magic, my only thought is Fuck it!

For the first time today, worms are not gnawing tunnels up my femur bones and out to the surface. Finally, I can take a full breath without feeling every joint creak. I feel normal, no longer dope sick. I am vaguely disappointed in myself for failing to follow through on my plan. Here I am again atop the levee with the sun setting, and I just blew almost sixteen hours of clean time. Well, not counting the oral spritz. The equipoise between the opiate swimming in my blood and the ongoing brain receptor catastrophe is soured by regret. I can't help feeling bad for shooting dope. My conscience is not happy. I wish I were more wasted, high enough to block the morose sense of dread.

Now not sweating or shaky, I can take my time and do it right. The remaining big vial of fentanyl is the reward I've sought. I stay in the vein on in my left arm and flood it with clear liquid fentanyl. The blue color washes out, chased pale up to my elbow. I rest my arm in my lap and let the drug pool in the veins of my extremity. Out slides the needle, and a tiny drop of blood grows at the point of injection. I put away the vial, syringes, and needles in the backpack, take a big breath, and bear down. I raise my hand up through the open roof and pump-squeeze my left fist in victory while the drug pours down my arm toward my heart. I feel the fentanyl hit my heart, then my lungs. A tide of calm. In twenty seconds a warm fleece blanket of joy and self-love spreads from deep inside my chest to engulf me completely.

The traffic outside seems to speed up. A snowy egret glowers at me before turning back to the muddy water and stabbing at a crayfish. For the moment, I have left everything behind. I am a boundless form dissolving into the universe. I have no past. The future is unimportant. All the little and large fires in my brain are snuffed out in the rising deluge of contentment the small fentanyl molecule affords. I am freer than free.

A vibration at my hip interrupts my freedom. The Motorola pager is set on escalate and the thrumming is getting more insistent. The number isn't the usual five digits we use in the hospital to contact each other. This number has seven digits, then a space, then four more. The four extra digits are a code for who sent the page. As a matter of custom, we send the five digits of the extension, then the final four digits of our own pager. The department was thoughtful enough to print and laminate a small card indexing everyone's pager number. I wore mine tethered neatly behind my name badge. Who could be paging me?

I look through the list, but it isn't one of my fellow residents. We get mistake pages sometimes. There is a voice recording played when you reach the pager's phone number. "Jason Giles, anesthesia," is my greeting, but people often don't listen for the audio and just set the receiver on the table when they dial. I have the surgery department laminated card, too. Looking down the columns—it isn't a surgeon who paged me. I should probably just call back, but I'd have to find a phone to do so. And I'm enjoying this moment too much.

Again, the pager buzzes and the window reads "1 msg." Same number and code. Not a mistake page. Fuck. I look over my anesthesia extension card again. Not a resident. Double checked and ruled out. I flip over the anesthesia card and look at the faculty list: 4838 – Peter G. Moore, Department Chair, Anesthesiology.

-4-
WHAT IS ADDICTION?

Addiction is defined many ways. Sometimes people describe it in terms of a drug or a behavior that they just can't stop doing. There is usually a suggestion of a compulsion or overwhelming desire to use a drug or to drink, even though the person knows drinking is bad for them. In the sobriety business, we talk about continued use despite adverse consequences, or doing something that hurts us, and we know it, but we do it anyway. This is where the idea of denial comes from. Denial posits the only way a person could possibly keep taking an addictive substance or engaging in an addictive behavior is if they're somehow not conscious of it. A glib, recovery cliché is the acronym for denial: Don't Even Notice I Am Lying. This is absurd. It's simply not possible to spend the kind of time and energy that most alcoholics or addicts spend getting/using the substance and dealing with the aftermath to not know it. So, let's just get rid of the idea of denial. It's silly.

I will allow that the deeper reasons – the backstory about how you got in trouble with drugs or alcohol – may not provide great insight or you may not want to talk about it, but that's not the same as not knowing that you have a problem. If you're reading this book for yourself, then you know you have a problem. If you're reading this book because you're worried about someone else, I hope we can answer those questions here. A recent Pew Poll reported 50 percent of Americans have a family member or close friend with a significant addiction problem. Let's spend a moment to define addiction.

Author, Steven Pressfield, who wrote one an excellent novel on the battle of Thermopylae, *The Gates of Fire*, lyrically describes the self-destructive, procrastinating demon we all have inside of us. Pressfield describes addiction as "activity without progress." That's one of my favorite definitions. Activity without progress describes a lot of us, doesn't it? Activity without progress is whirling around, careening from situation to situation. Promises welched upon, hearts broken, missed opportunities, blown-off connections, skipped success at work, wrecked relationships, and lots of jumping around without getting anywhere are common "tells" of addiction.

From a biological standpoint, addiction is described by the Substance Abuse and Mental Health Agency (SAMHSA) as a "brain disease or a brain disorder." I question that description because it isn't especially helpful. Addiction is not a disease. We talk about disease in medicine as an entity or pathologic process that we can treat with medicine, surgery, energy (e.g. radiation), or behavior therapy. The most obvious example is a disease like an infection.

Take pneumonia, for example. If you go to the doctor with a cough, fever, and feeling lousy, she will order a chest X-ray that may reveal an infection in your lung. If so, she will typically prescribe you antibiotics, which kill bacteria. With the bacteria gone, you'll return to a normal state and the pneumonia will be gone. But when medical people describe addiction as a disease, they describe it in terms of a chronic condition. Addiction is often compared with diabetes or high blood pressure.

You probably already know, diabetes and high blood pressure are physiologic conditions marked by elevated blood glucose, or high blood pressure readings, respectively. High blood sugar is the hallmark of diabetes, but it is not the cause, it's just an indicator we follow. The real problem likely has something to do with special cells in the pancreas or the liver cells. Science hasn't answered that question yet. We aren't sure how a person's sugar metabolism is messed up. Since we can't follow what we don't understand, we follow the glucose.

In the case of a person with addiction, addiction doctors pay attention to behavior. We examine how much they drink, of course. We also follow physiologic markers and look for evidence of damage caused by alcohol (or drugs). For example, blood counts or liver function lab tests can shed light on the severity of body damage from alcohol exposure. Whether you have a drinking/drug problem, you still have the same old ordinary problems everyone else has. The same brain deals with the ordinary stresses of life: avoiding death, finding food, finding a mate, getting shelter, reproduction, trying to live a life with meaning. All those processes are still in place whether a person has addiction or not.

One way to think about addiction is like a hijacker of your normal mental processes, steering you to places you don't want to go. The best way I heard that described was by a friend of mine, Jerry. He used to have a problem with heroin. Jerry describes the process like a thief breaking into a house. The first thing the thief does is disable the alarm system. That's a good way to think about addiction. Altered judgment is the consequence of the chemical's effect on the physical matter of the brain (and its function of thinking). But that still doesn't mean the person is diseased.

Travel with me to the past for a moment to frame the disease question in an historical context. Wine and beer have been integral to the diet and culture of man prior to recorded history. A clay jar discovered in modern day Georgia, near Russia, contained the dregs of wine produced in 8000 B.C. We know the ancient Egyptians drank beer. An outlier for his time, Alexander the Great, died of acute alcohol poisoning (mead). When the Romans conquered Greece, they adopted the more moderate drinking habits of the vanquished. Essentially, all the alcohol consumed by humans through the Renaissance is some form of wine or beer. Many attempts at distillation are recorded before the 16th century in far-flung places like India, China, and Mesoamerica, but with no way to cool the ethanol vapor, the resulting concentration of alcohol remained around 5 to 10 percent.

Chemists began synthesizing aqua vitae in volume in the 17th century. With alcohol concentrations of up to 90 percent, the "spirit" of the wine was concentrated. It was available at the chemist – today we would say the pharmacy – and it was doled out sparingly. Distillation equipment (the origin of the word still) was at the time made of glass, then expensive to produce. Copper pot stills were much less costly and became widely available in a new nation. Early Americans had only the rudiments of infrastructure. Moving raw material over long distances incurred high transit costs. Rural grain farmers could convert their harvest into much more portable distilled spirits. Stills were spotted on nearly every farm in western Pennsylvania by Dr. Benjamin Rush, during a trip to Carlisle in 1784.

Dr. Rush was one of the first to equate drinking spirits with the development of physical diseases. He favored the heavy taxation of whisky, a policy that when implemented led to the Whisky Rebellion. By 1791 the new government was in debt to France and Spain and needed to raise tax revenue. Distilled spirits were the first item taxed by Congress, and the Pennsylvania farmers refused to pay it in 1794. Washington himself would lead a militia of thirteen thousand troops, but there was no conflict as the five hundred farmers, who'd earlier burned down the taxman's house, all went home. Jefferson repealed the whisky tax ten years later. By the year of his death in 1799, Washington was the largest distiller of spirits in Virginia.

Whisky consumption (and other distilled spirits) continued to grow through the 19th century, peaking at seven and a half gallons of pure alcohol per person per year (ppy) in 1830 (today it is around two gallons ppy). Together with this rise in consumption, mostly by men, came a rise in the temperance movement; it was largely a response by the wives of the inebriates. In America, two major social tides and a civil war set the trajectory for reform. The Second Great Awakening, the rise of Unitarianism over Calvinism, and the Union victory over the Confederate states each helped consolidate the idea that excess of consumption of alcohol was a sin. Louder came the calls that this sin should be stamped out by the government.

The 19th Amendment to the Constitution (prohibition of alcohol manufacture and sale) and woman's suffrage both became national laws in 1920. Until repeal in 1933, people still got drunk, but they mostly bought their alcohol from the black market "bootleggers." Anyone who became dependent on alcohol was regarded as a social outcast.

These helpless souls were gross depictions of sin incarnate. Medicine came to the rescue, at least in nomenclature. Dr. Rush's idea that alcohol caused disease was repackaged to "alcohol drinking is the disease," and that disease was so-named alcoholism. Not to worry though, science was soon about to save the alcoholic with new medicines and therapies. They included belladonna, morphine, electroshock therapy, and in severe cases, frontal lobotomy. If science wasn't successful with curing alcoholism it wasn't for lack of zeal.

Before the 1950s, most of America still considered people who drank too much, or who took drugs, as having weak willpower or a moral failing. The American Medical Association issued a statement in 1956 recognizing alcoholism as an illness. By 1966 it was rechristened a disease. This followed the increased profile of Alcoholics Anonymous in the Oscar-winning film The Lost Weekend.

With the rise of AA, there excess drinking was held up not as a failure of morality or willpower, but rather as an illness or a mental disease. At the same time, the rise of psychiatry through the works of Sigmund Freud, Carl Jung, B.F. Skinner, and others, offered new hope for curing the alcoholic once and for all. Pharma would produce a string of medications specifically aimed at altering mood or behavior, especially the anxiety that at the time was believed to cause alcoholism.

The 1966 Rolling Stones hit Mother's Little Helper highlights the effect of Valium, introduced in 1963. Marketed by Roche as a miracle drug, doctors were armed with several "non-addicting" medications to combat the problem of alcohol. The definition of disease was expanded further and eventually included habits of every variety. It is not an improvement in the arena of self-determination to be told that you don't have a moral failing or a weak will, but instead you have a disease. More, you have a brain disease. A mental disease. It's hard for me to see how this is an improvement.

In the 21st century we have incredibly sophisticated tools for studying brain activity. We can scan the brain and see how individual areas are functioning from a metabolic standpoint. A test called an fMRI reveals which parts of the brain are more active than others. The images produced are amazing and vividly show elegant details, but you still can't tell what a person is thinking. If anyone tells you he understands how the brain works, he's pulling your leg. We haven't fully illuminated the normal brain, much less the "chemically imbalanced one." We are like the early explorers: Columbus before funding from Queen Isabella, standing on the Spanish coast, looking westward.

Persistent, though, is this stubborn concept of disease. Employing the disease concept naturally opens the door to treatment with medication and hospitalization. The concept was promoted because something had to be done to help those so afflicted. I get it, but we know more now. The addiction process resides far deeper and more fundamentally than the term disease defines. It is in how all of us are put together. In Steven Quartz and Anette Asp's book Cool: How the Brain's Hidden Quest for Cool Drives Our Economy and Shapes Our World, they describe three types of value judgment systems. The first system is goal-directed, the next is the survival system, and the last one is habit or routine.

If you look at addiction using their model of brain function – a mixture of goals, habits, and the survival instinct – you'll get a better version of how the normal processes of the brain are a bit out of whack in the addict. Much of addiction is no more than habit or routine. In times past, we used to call drug or alcohol dependence a habit, and with good reason. Much of ongoing drug and alcohol use is simply because it has become a routine. We did the same thing yesterday – or ten times earlier today. It becomes like second nature.

If you follow the news, you know addiction claims hundreds of lives every day. It kills more people in the U.S. than car crashes do. The opiate crisis grips America, and the whole field of mental health, especially in addiction medicine, is desperately trying to solve this problem. Calling it a brain disease may seem like a trivial matter – the way it's always been done – but framing the problem correctly makes an enormous difference. Characterizing people who drink too much or use drugs as normal people, but with a perturbed or upset pattern of thinking, is far better than calling them diseased. It's not just semantics, but rather a more accurate model of addiction itself. There is a vast difference in openness and willingness to change, between telling someone he must change his habits, and diagnosing him a mental disease. Treatment should be aimed at changing the way a person thinks and feels about himself. We are generally bad at accurately assessing ourselves. Alcoholics and drug addicts are neither diseased nor defective, per se. They have a well-established, albeit self-destructive, habit pattern.

Neither should addiction be glibly defined as a chemical imbalance. If it were, that would imply that the brain is static and unchanging. Clearly the brain is dynamic and incredibly adaptive. It's also exceptionally good at adjusting to reality moment to moment. On the fly. Saying you have too much of one brain chemical, a neurotransmitter like dopamine for example, or too little of another one, like GABA, is simplistic to the extreme. Let me explain this in a little more detail, for it is vital to understanding what addiction is and is not.

Case in point: opioids. In the same breath, addiction professionals speak of chemical imbalance and the phenomenon of tolerance when describing the effects of opioids on the brain. They admit the brain adapts to Vicodin but not to dopamine or GABA (or Seroquel). Inconsistent, right? Remember your favorite restaurant, the place that was so amazing when you first went there, but after years of eating the same meal, has the cuisine lost some luster? We naturally adapt to almost anything.

The worst part about the "chemical imbalance" version of the brain is that it gives the impression that we know more than we really do. I think it's much more productive to look at how people behave. If we pay attention, we will notice patterns in the way people habituated to substances tend to act. Counterintuitive self-sabotaging behaviors are remarkably similar between people, regardless of their addiction picture.

In summary, addiction isn't a disease. It is a complex interplay of ancient neural automation and a present-day stressful environment. The same neurodevelopmental miracles that made humans the top organism on the planet also have their downsides. We automate behavior and we use tools to change the environment. One set of tools is mind-altering chemicals. The environment upon which they act is our internal milieu. Man, attempting to manage all he sees, naturally manages himself and his moods if he can. Unfortunately, in this regard, we are built to form habits. Self-destructive routine development is the proper place to apply our efforts toward relieving addiction, not further alienating and "pathologizing" a normal process.

☐

-5-

HABITS

What did you do this morning right after you woke up? 80% of people check their smartphone within fifteen minutes of waking. Most of these within five minutes of opening their eyes. Phone done, ok. Now, after checking your messages, did you jump in the shower, brush your teeth? Did you lie in bed and meditate, or did you get on your knees and pray? Maybe you flipped on the TV? Or maybe you pulled the covers up over your head.

Our morning routine sets the tone for the day. Bit by bit we add to our startup rituals. Mine involves a cup of coffee, unless I'm on a tea jag. Morning routine components are hard to discard as well. Try plugging I your phone in another part of the house overnight. Most people get anxious even thinking about it.

This begs a question, "Can we program ourselves to take constructive actions rather than drift along as slaves to old habits?" Scott Adams, creator of the beloved workplace cartoon Dilbert, wrote a book called How To Fail At Pretty Much Everything And Still Be A Success. Adams recounts his life as a cog in the giant corporate machine for years, how he started the cartoon, and how to build a talent stack. It's a funny title, but the message from the book is sound: our brains are like wet computers. We can program them with specific information and they will execute the instructions faithfully–just like a smartphone. Now, like all computers, there can be faults, and some programs are harder to write than others. But, in general, our brains are best at repetitive activities.

Another angle on the same subject is found in the book *Cool, How the Brain's Hidden Quest for Cool Drives Our Economy and Shapes Our World*, by Steven Quartz and Annette Asp. The Cal Tech professors discourse eloquently on the organization of brain systems into task units. The energy-saving evolutionary blockbuster advantage we have over all other animals: repetition. We do things over and over because automation dramatically decreases brain processing power. And we are better at it than any creature that walks the earth. Accounting for only two percent of body weight, our brain consumes roughly twenty percent of our calorie intake. We have a multi-core processor running our body and perception sensing systems, but at enormous metabolic cost.

Evolution, never satisfied with merely good design (as found in our simian relatives), improved the automatic functions in us. We're so good at it, that wherever possible, the brain will automate any regular routine to minimize work load.

The brain can process sixty quadrillion bits of information per second; data from your eyes alone are over forty-seven million bits per second. If you could give your full attention to all data that just your eyes handle, your brain would have to be about one hundred times larger than it is. Most of the light processed by our retinas and optic nerves into brain signals is ignored because it is irrelevant to us. We are selective in our attention, and where possible we automate even our attention focus.

"Excellence is an art won by training and habituation. We do not act rightly because we have virtue or excellence, but rather we have those because we have acted rightly. We are what we repeatedly do. Excellence, then, is not an act but a habit." Aristotle, Poetics.

———

The ancient Greeks understood habit was the key to success. It is also the key to failure. In the 20th century, you'd hear alcoholism or tobacco dependence referred to as 'a drinking habit' or 'a smoking habit'. In our quest for control of the mind, we have become more precise but less accurate. We speak about chemical imbalance and wounded inner-children and we've drifted away from a more sound and defensible concept: habit. Substance-use-as habit is still valid and more useful as ever. Drugs or no, we perfect our actions with time and repetition. Instead of peeling the onion's layers, let's talk about dicing them.

When I first learned to chop an onion, I was terrible at it. I was eighteen years old and though I had poor manual dexterity. My onion often rolled off the island. I hacked it at ugly angles; more than once I cut myself. Pile on sulfurous fumes wafting up from the cut edged, my nose ran and I cried a lot. Onion chopping was a challenge for me when I first went at one in the kitchen. Not long after, I became an apprentice prep cook in a very fancy Italian restaurant.

I was taught by *Hell's Kitchen* judge chef Josie Le Balch how to properly chop an onion. After countless hours of practice as a prep cook, I eventually got the hang of vegetables. Though I never got to Josie's level, I'm not an amateur slicer either. The main difference after her teaching and my practice is I stopped thinking about each small knife and onion movement.

While learning to dice, I concentrated on details at millimeter scale. As my proficiency grew, I thought less about how, and more about consistency of the final product. Connections between nerve cells—synapses—are how habit loops are formed. The brain is constantly changing and can form new habit loops if we live. Once we make a habit loop, they are remarkably stable and near impossible to undo.

Do you remember learning to drive a car? Each small turn of the steering wheel, or slight press down on the gas pedal demanded your full attention. Learning to drive is exhausting. With practice, we develop a habit of the small adjustments and we're free to focus on the journey. Distracted driving keeps us from using our habit loops efficiently, as well as pulling our attention away from the road.

Let's look a little more closely at Aristotle's quote. He is talking about excellence, standing above. Weirdly, most who have substance habits are exceptionally proficient in some skill. It's almost as if the talent gene were inherited along with the alcoholism gene. Alcoholism, as you know, is multifactorial: so is talent. Still, they seem to be co-inherited.

Excellence is something we all strive for; it provides material rewards and elevated social status. Aristotle thought pursuit of excellence itself was an art. He also told is exactly how to achieve excellence. It is won by training and habituation. Training is precisely what you're undergoing now – training for how to live life free from the bondage of drugs and alcohol. Habituation is the second key needed to unlock the art of excellence. We not only train our minds and bodies for maximal effort and accomplishment, but practice doing so repeatedly until we've created an automatic routine. A habit of excellence.

Regarding spirituality, Aristotle says humans do not intrinsically have virtue. We develop virtue when we repeatedly act rightly. Life is in the doing; the existentialists are right. We are not passive subjects in an imperial regime. We have agency, are engineered for action, and our actions are the beams and joists of a life of meaning. Our conduct determines our harvest: excellence or detritus.

There's redemption as well as judgment in Aristotle's remarks. Since we are what we repeatedly do, we should be careful what we develop proficiency in. If you regularly lie, if you skip opportunities to be useful to others, if you shirk your work, neglect your body, your family, and if you do this over a considerable period, you will still become what you repeatedly do.

Most people who have a weight problem didn't get that way all at once. They have an established set of habits and patterns that lead to more caloric intake daily than their bodies expend. Habits can be accounted for in caloric overage, but it is the routine that causes problems. In fact, the obesity is a side effect of the two things in this case: proficiency at consuming more calories than you need daily, and the consistent habit of doing it every day.

Let's be honest, habitual drug use follows the same pattern. In my case, I didn't intend to develop substance dependence; no way did I want to become a fentanyl addict. Yet, my small but consistent routine of drug use was focused on getting and staying loaded. I started small, one day at a time, and eventually I was proficient with injectable opioids. As my skills acquiring and administering the drug improved, I thought less and less about the details and more and more about using the tool (fentanyl) to manage my inner life. The threads of habit are too weak to be felt until they're too strong to be broken.

The clever and sophisticated brain is masterful at consolidating routine. It perfects habits even if we aren't paying much attention. Some folks can carry on a covert opioid habit far longer than I did. I lasted less than a year grappling with powerful narcotics. I know men and women who hung on for far longer, but at a tremendous personal cost. The brain knows almost no limits in its ability to form and maintain habits. The most talented musicians show us what habit can accomplish and what it can destroy.

Prince fell victim to the same drug which almost killed me: fentanyl. The world lost his brilliance in 2016; one of the greatest musicians of all time. Pull up the YouTube of the Beatles', "While my Guitar Gently Weeps," the recording with the guitar solo Prince plays at the end of the song. He transcends playing the guitar and moves into unconscious communication with the audience.

Prince isn't thinking about each note he touches. He wraps his listeners and bandmates in unrequited longing, and never hesitates over the next note. He is not thinking about specific finger pressure, how lightly to press or how much to bend a note. Prince exemplified Aristotle's vision of excellence. Habit giveth, and habit taketh away.

There are diverse estimates of how long it takes to develop a new habit. A definition repeated most often comes from Dr. Maxwell Maltz, a plastic surgeon writing in the 1930s. Maltz observed his patients took up to sixty-six days to accept their new appearance following surgery, with the average being around twenty-one days. Twenty-one days is a wonderful bite-sized little nugget for the self-help.

Dr. Maltz was interested in changing the self-concept, whether by affirmation or scalpel. The fallacy of three weeks to a new you, reinforces the feeling sense of worthlessness and failure. Others master a new habit in twenty-one days, *what's the matter with you?* It feels tantalizingly close; all we need to do is exert some effort. We want credit for our intentions.

Some habits are easier to establish than others. Habits requiring complex preparation, elaborate sequences of action, or a lot of mental processing are more difficult to get going. Simple ones, like drinking a glass of water when you wake up, are much easier to initiate. But easy to do is also easy not to do. Besides setting ourselves up to act, we need to make it automatic to continue a new habit. We can prime ourselves for success in the water example, by having some ready to go on the nightstand before we go to sleep.

Stanford professor BJ Fogg, in his book *Tiny Habits*, recommends flossing just one tooth to kick off the habit of better dental hygiene. Small wins are the underlying mechanism of the one-tooth-strategy. If you can do one, regularly, you can establish the habit. One leads to two which leads to your whole smile.

Deeper explorations of the time required to establish a new habit reveal the heavy influence of social cues. Addiction recovery lore says is you'll need ninety days to establish a new (sober) habit. Alcoholics Anonymous' standard advice to the newcomer is he should attend ninety meetings in ninety days.

There is no empirical evidence to support this duration or frequency of meeting attendance, nor is there much data to support that meeting attendance by itself makes that much of a difference. Nevertheless, there are good data that suggest people who have remained sober typically develop a stable, supportive social environment where they can discuss their current problems. A social group of peers multiplies your joys and divides your sorrows, if you are a regular participant.

'Ninety in ninety' is a dogma and it's worth a few minutes of closer inspection. Besides how much we love alliteration and rhyme, three consecutive months is a significant and sustained period of effort. You don't have to go to *a meeting a day*, but the implication is you should. Daily repetition of a complex sobriety-focused set of actions produces a change in salience. We come to believe a sober life is possible and we experience by our own actions said life is within reach. We endow our actions with meaning because they're ours.

Two elements of a ninety-in-ninety sidebar recommendation are: 1) sustained effort of attending a meeting every day and, 2) the influence this routine has on the rest of your daily schedule. Establishment of a new routine is the goal. Drinking or using habits cannot be abolished; their habit loops are permanent too. We build more automatic habits that carry us through. Author James Clear says we don't rise to the level of our goals, but we fall to the level of our systems (habits).

If every evening at seven o'clock you attend a meeting of Alcoholics

Anonymous, then it will in time become established habit. People at the meeting will come to expect you there, and you'll likely make friends and maybe even to do things together outside of the meeting rooms of the fellowship. Maybe get a cup of coffee.

Even if this doesn't happen, blocking out of your schedule at a regular time to attend a meeting will have consequences on the rest of your day. You'll simply have to get things done before going to the meeting, and putting yourself in the mindset of doing them is beneficial itself. You will not only accomplish the tasks that you have been putting off, but you will feel more effective in your life. This is the opposite of unmanageability and how you'll feel keeping your word to yourself is worth far more than the effort you'll put in to keep your word.

There is tremendous benefit simply making a commitment to a routine. When we decide that we are going to do something, there is a supernova of energy released. William Murray's (often misattributed to Goethe) quote comes to mind:

"Until one is committed, there is hesitancy, the chance to draw back. Concerning all acts of initiative (and creation), there is one elementary truth, the ignorance of which kills countless ideas and splendid plans: that the moment one definitely commits oneself, then Providence moves too. All sorts of things occur to help one that would never otherwise have occurred. A whole stream of events issues from the decision, raising in one's favor all manner of unforeseen incidents and meetings and material assistance, which no man could have dreamed would have come his way. Whatever you can do, or dream you can do, begin it. Boldness has genius, power, and magic in it. Begin it now."

I first learned Dr. Murray's quote as a teenager, and I have continued to learn from it since. There is something beyond understanding which flows from commitment. If you'll make a commitment to go to ninety meetings in ninety days, or to keep track of your alcohol intake, or to tell the truth no matter what, you will experience an internal shift. Your identity will change from a person who founders to one who sails straight and far across the deep oceans of life.

When we commit to something, when we put our sense of integrity and our word on the line, we always pay a little extra attention, put a little more effort and we are far less likely to give up on ourselves. Another quote, this one from Jules Renard, was good enough to be placed on a road sign in in

India:

"Laziness is nothing more than the habit of resting before you're tired."

Give yourself a chance to get tired through effort, and commit to changing your life. Focusing on commitment will make a huge difference. Take your commitment further and do what Ben Franklin did and write it down.

Jordan Peterson released a program designed to help you gain mastery of your self-discipline called "Self-Authoring." You can find it at jordanbpeterson.com, under a tab with the same label. Self-authoring is no more complicated than writing a story about yourself in the present, future, and past. This is like the experience of being in a room of Alcoholics Anonymous and telling your story. Saying aloud your thoughts and fears, allowing them out of your own head, so you can hear what you sound like is priceless. Double the value when you hear your (sometimes) whacky thoughts reflected in the comments of others. This will give you a new perspective. Self-authoring's goal is to change the story you tell yourself.

It's far more than a goal-setting exercise, or an autobiographical review of major epochs in your life. Focusing on what you think about yourself can yield tremendous benefits. We each carry around in our minds our story. Our ideals, goals, and moral guidelines of conduct. We feel worst when we transgress our own morals, and we feel best when we strive toward our highest ideal. Dr. Peterson would say, without a purpose, our lives are not only meaningless but they drift aimlessly. A purpose is a rudder with which to steer the ship of our lives.

When I began surgery training, I was not very good at tying knots. Surgical knots must be precise, for they are essential to create the proper tension to close an incision. Sutures are also the preferred method of attaching an object (like a drainage tube) temporarily to the skin. They hold securely in a way that tape can't. And once cut, they're easy to remove. During an operation, surgeons must insure the sutures are correctly tied, efficiently and in a consistent manner.

I fumbled with the thin thread, my surgical gloves hampering my clumsy knot-tying in the slippery operative field. I needed to improve in a hurry. After the case, the surgeon suggested I get a pack of surgical suture material to practice tying knots.

To start I was all thumbs. Often I lost track which direction I put down the first knot and would tie a "granny" (slipknot). The loops and tails caught on my fingers as I tried to pull them through the hole. It is worth a quick look on the Internet to see how to tie proper surgical knots. It's an elegant little move done thousands of times a day around the world by surgeons. Experienced surgeons can tie a knot with only one hand.

Black and heavy, number zero silk is also cheap and plentiful in a hospital. I always had a pack of silk with me. I got into the *habit* of tying knots everywhere I went: on the zipper of my backpack, on the steering wheel of my car as I drove, on the handle of the shopping cart in the supermarket.

I tied thousands and thousands of knots. I found my rhythm, and passed from novice to adept. I started using my left hand because sometimes the angle during surgery requires you to use the opposite hand to get the knot down in correct orientation.

I practiced, practiced, and practiced more until I got very good. Eventually when I was in a case and my professor wanted me to place a knot in a specific spot, I could do so with the right tension, direction, and orientation. Tying a knot became second nature. After thousands of tiny macramé links left in heavy black silk thread on countless chair backs, I'd mastered the moves. No longer consciously thinking how to do it; my hands did it automatically. I could even tie one-handed knots.

In writing this story, I wondered if I still remembered how to tie the knots. I got out some black thread Dr. Giles keeps in her sewing kit. I cut a length, wrapped it around the handle of my desk drawer, and automatically my hands started tying knots again. It was as if no time had passed between when I last tied them., the sub-routine is not only automated, but it's still in my brain.

———

William James, in his classic book Habit, sketched out a lifelong process:

"The hell to be endured hereafter, of which theology tells, is no worse than the hell we make for ourselves in this world by habitually fashioning our characters in the wrong way. Could the young but realize how soon they will become mere walking bundles of habits, they would give more heed to their conduct while in the plastic state.

We are spinning our fates, good or evil, and never to be undone. Every smallest stroke of virtue or of vice leaves its never-so-little scar. The drunken Rip Van Winkle, in Jefferson's play, excuses himself for every fresh dereliction by saying, 'I won't count this time!" Well! He may not count it, and a kind Heaven may not count it; but it is being counted none the less. Down among his nerve-cells and fibers the molecules are counting it, registering and storing it up to be used against him when the next temptation comes.

Nothing we ever do is, in strict scientific literalness, wiped out. Of course this has its good side as well as its bad one. As we become permanent drunkards by so many separate drinks, so we become saints in the moral, and authorities and experts in the practical and scientific spheres, by so many separate acts and hours of work. Let no youth have any anxiety about the upshot of his education, whatever the line of it may be. If he keeps faithfully busy each hour of the working-day, he may safely leave the final result to itself. He can with perfect certainty count on waking up some fine morning, to find himself one of the competent ones of his generation, in whatever pursuit he may have singled out."

In 1891 when Dr. James wrote this passage, there was no such thing as an MRI machine. He didn't know about dopamine or neural development. And yet, when he speaks about "programming that leaves the never-so-little scars," he's describing the permanent molecular changes of habit. The good thing about automating processes is when we create a habit that helps us, like tying a surgical knot, they remain forever, literally, at our fingertips. Unfortunately, the automated tendencies toward self-destructive negative and bad habits are also permanently etched in the neural architecture of the brain.

This also explains why even after a long period of abstinence from drinking or drug use, when someone returns to substance use, the existing habit loop springs into action. The classic outcome: quickly our man finds himself in very bad shape. Time away from an active substance habit loop does not lead to its atrophy. Like old machinery, covered with tarps or dust cloths, we fire up the old habit loops when we return to substance use. We are usually stunned how quickly we get back to where we left off.

If you go to Alcoholics Anonymous, you might hear a colloquial expression about your brain after a period of abstinence. Something like, "your disease is doing push-ups while you're not drinking (using)". I applaud the insight about habits: they're definitely resident in the brain. The good folks in A.A. though are wrong to imply a habit loop is *strengthened* without ongoing activation/use. But I agree with the concept of picking up where you left off. Time abstinent from substances builds new, and one hopes better, habits. The old ones are still there though. The speed with which even a long-time sober person can plunge back into the depths of substance debauchery is impressive. But please, let's stop with the push-ups.

Also, the sub-conscious habits of acquiring, using, and recovering from the aftereffects (hangover) of drug and alcohol intoxication are typically so automatic they are part of a larger habit-loop complex. Like a cassette tape or CD, they're "played" through the mechanism of routines and actions. Once the neurological 'play' button is pushed, we obey these habit-loops without thinking. Memorialized by the cliché, "It's like riding a bicycle, once you know how you never forget." Bike riding is another everyday example of automated neural processing.

Malcolm Gladwell, in his book, Outliers, floats the concept of ten thousand hours of an activity to achieve mastery. Proficiency or habit occurs with far fewer hours of practice. One of the more interesting examples given is of the British pop group The Beatles. They played together in clubs around Liverpool, but it was when they took a long-term gig in Germany they got good. Gladwell calculates the Fab Four spent ten thousand hours together. They countlessly repeated their songs, learned the subtleties of each band member's style, and harmonized together.

Their efforts have endured almost sixty years. They remain beloved as the most successful and famous music group of all time. Their music also has a timeless quality and a global appeal which are unmatched.

Ten thousand abstinent hours is 417 days. If you can put together a habit sequence that long, you've got a great shot at keeping abstinent if you desire. The day-to-day routine of not drinking becomes a new (and eventually automatic) habit. Not drinking or using, even when you feel like it, are also skills. Like any other habit, if you practice them with dedication and for the long-haul, you'll create stable good habits which will see you through challenging times.

Jon Acuff, in his book *Finish*, describes goal setting from a different perspective. If you're like me, perfectionism is a habit I wish I didn't have. Steven Pressfield calls it out as part of your intrinsic resistance to surrendering your work product. The perfectionist has no deadline for submission.

If I can't accomplish something superlative, I tend to say, "Fuck it." As pertains to beating a substance habit, when emotional challenges, boredom or alienation overwhelm, it is not unusual to seek comfort in a previous coping strategy. We dig through the dustbin looking for a way that worked in the past. Exhibit A of the "fuck it" strategy is going back to drinking or using when something bad happens to you.

We all make poor decisions under duress. The urgent swamps the important. Our imperative is get out of pain now. It's unlikely we'll muster the courage to stick with the don't-use plan. In fact, relapse to substance use is so common, in the rehab world you'll hear the expression "Relapse is part of recovery."

I know many struggling souls who, following a brief relapse, then stayed away from their recovery community for years; they were too embarrassed to come back and admit that they had slipped. This must end. I shudder speculate on how many have died tormented by the idea they've failed. It's hard to make a new habit, and we shouldn't shame anyone who has the courage to try.

More than just in A.A., the failure connoted by relapse seeps into family structures, friend groups, and work relationships. Believing you should be "cured," especially after a few weeks in rehab, is comical. All humans veer toward addiction, the habitual soothing of anxiety and discomfort. Doing so is as natural as the sunrise, and just as predictable. Attempting to control your own behavior, seeking healthy and sustainable ways of dealing with stress—in short, growing up—should be celebrated. This is true even if it takes you several attempts before your new habit sticks. You haven't failed to change until you quit trying. You need only work to be successful today. Let tomorrow take care of itself. Let's not borrow trouble from the future.

Living life one day at a time is a useful strategy. We free ourselves from overanxious concerns that won't ever come to pass. But sometimes a whole day is too much. It's perfectly acceptable to break up the twenty-four into smaller parts. Some days I say to myself, "one morning at a time." Or a quarter of an hour on extra-rough days. When first sober, committing to a *whole day* of abstinence was, sometimes, too much to tackle. I'd bargain with the "committee" in my head just to stay sober until lunch. I'd let after-noon Jason decide about the rest of the day.

I would ask myself, *can you make it till noon?* If the answer was no, I would negotiate, *how about until 10 A.M.?* That was only a couple of hours away. I can make it two hours. Dr. James described the habitual drunkard as the accumulation of countless drinks over years. Likewise, the habitual sober person is the accumulation of multiple refusals over a considerable time.

If you have slipped, or relapsed, don't despair. Making a new habit is hard. Just like when you learn to ride a bike, you crash a lot before figuring it out. It's not easy to acquire the skill of coordinated balance while steering an unstable, two-wheel vehicle. The same thing is true for sobriety, only it's way harder than riding a bike.

There are emotional and environmental snares, below your conscious awareness, to pull you back to the quick relief of picking up a substance. Automated, steel-cable-strong habits compiled over years, collaborate to make sliding backwards feel inevitable. Take change in small actions; reach out and ask for help often. If you're using the VHAB app, stay connected to your community as often as you like. We don't pretend to be stoically superhuman. We all have feet of clay. If we can right ourselves when we stumble, and stick with the plan, we'll be okay.

Surgeon Dr. Atul Gawande, in *The Checklist Manifesto*, beautifully outlines the staying on track as you build a new habit. Hired by the World Health Organization to reduce worldwide surgical infection rates, his task seemed herculean. How could one surgeon change the behavior of thousands of others scattered globally over one hundred fifty countries? With hospital systems as diverse as those in Calcutta, Geneva, and Houston, how could one man make reduce post-op infection rates? Doctor Gawande wisely began by looking at the habits of surgeons.

Dr. G's insight into human behavior, especially the power of forming new habits, is worth a read. His tangible goal was lowering the rate of surgical infections. He found two key clinical decision points which make a big difference in outcome.

First is the timing of intravenous antibiotics. If you have surgery, the anesthesiologist gives you I.V. antibiotics an hour before incision. Being imperfect, we can get a little off schedule.

If the antibiotics are given too early before surgery, they're cleared from the body and can't kill bacteria. They must be circulating in your skin when the scalpel cuts. The cul-de-sac of a hair follicle harbors bacteria; topical disinfectant (iodine, alcohol) can't get down to the base of the hair. If the antibiotics are administered after the operation, they don't do as much good. Blood supply is restricted near the operative site because the little blood vessels have been cut. Bacteria dragged into the wound by the incision are now free to multiply, infect and kill you. With infections responsible for a lot of post-surgical deaths, morbidity, and cost, reducing them is a top priority.

Second, nurses seemed uncomfortable reminding the surgeons and anesthesiologists to administer the antibiotics on time. Gawande believed surgeons resented erosion of their authority when subordinates "gave orders" to the Big Kahuna. I disagree with his explanation; Gawande himself found most nurses were unconcerned about vestigial MD/RN hierarchy. Nurses are vigorous patient advocates. The low-hanging fruit of change: make and follow a checklist.

People get distracted and they forget to complete mundane tasks–like giving pre-op antibiotics. Gawande imposed a checklist on himself and his operating room team. He helped everyone stay on track and create new automated habits. Infection and death rates fell by 35%. The two-minute checklist has become standard worldwide. The lesson: a checklist holds you accountable to your intentions. The result for the W.H.O. was a global reduction in surgical infection

I think of the checklist as analogous to the slalom flags on a downhill skiing course. You can ski wherever you want to, but if you go back and forth through the gates, then you will stay on the trail. If you don't pass a gate for some time, then you're probably off the trail, and you may be headed for danger. Off the side of a mountain, is not a good place to find yourself out in the snow.

Lao Tzu wrote, "The faintest ink is better than the best memory." The checklist converts the challenge of remembering a new routine it into simply following some instructions to reach your goal. Checklists are not orders from headquarters or to-do lists. They're tools to nudge our memory. Memory and judgment are intrinsically shaky, and a checklist keeps us on track. In the process of recovery, we can easily forget the simple things: don't use substances, ask for help, show up tell the truth.

Checklists are short and simple reminders of what we need to do. They promote self-discipline and encourage creativity. If you follow their order and do what you set out to, your ability to execute on your commitments will improve. Remember, checklists are not magic. If you don't do what you're supposed to do, if you don't take care of yourself then a checklist isn't going to save you. If you've done everything you're supposed to do on your checklist but you still feel crummy, then you need a better checklist.

Following a checklist offers another benefit. They help us to recognize deeper patterns of behavior and habit. You might experience internal resistance to putting something on your checklist that you know will make a difference. We keep a stash of excuses for why we don't change. Checklists are unyielding judges of our actions. They help us take an honest look at our actions. The unexamined life, as Socrates said, is not worth living.

To recap, human beings are a triumph of habit formation. We have automated processes, or habit loops, which allow us to use our considerable brain power on something besides the minute to minute focused fixation on activity. Unfortunately, bad habits – the automated process of self-destructive behaviors – is also a natural consequence of how our brains are constructed. Instead of fighting the magic of habit formation, we can use checklists and reminders to harvest its power.

–6–

HOW MY HABIT STARTED
–AND ENDED

One of the must-see destinations on the west coast, Santa Monica, is a bustling city of entertainment, technology, and tourism. Now nicknamed silicon beach, the seaside town supports Google and hundreds of other

Internet companies. In the 1970s, when I was a kid, the city was still substantially industrial.

I lived in a rent-controlled apartment in the working-class part of town with my mother, dad, and younger sister. Here's what my life was like back then.

My dad drinks every day. The older I get, the more obvious it is he can't go a day without a cocktail. He tries many times to stop drinking. Eventually, he stops for good, but this happens in 1985. Most often, he goes missing after a screaming match with my mother. As my sister and I grow older, he'll fight with one or both of us. He is unsettled and dissatisfied with himself but he takes that out on his nuclear family. Curt Giles drinks to smother feelings of self-dissatisfaction. He's stands six feet three and tips the scale over two hundred pounds. He used to come home from bar fights with banged-up knuckles. We all try not to make him mad. You get the picture.

I fix him a drink at the same time every afternoon, three o'clock, because I get home from elementary school at 2:45 and he doesn't go to work until just before five. He drinks Gilbey's gin on the rocks, or Beefeater for variety. I twist the plastic tray and remove four translucent cubes and drop them in a bucket glass. If the bottle is new, I slit the blue tax seal with my thumbnail before twisting off the cap.

I listen to the crackle of the cubes as the warmer liquid makes them swell and fracture. I feel powerful mixing up his medicine. A couple of drinks in him and he's much easier to be around. No drinks at all is bad. Jumpy. Irritated. Mean. More than four is bad also. Over-affectionate. Maudlin. Sad. There is a sweet spot, though. A dose where he was kind but not cruel. We pass through this spot every afternoon on the way to Mopeytown.

Tuesday nights, my sister and I go to Al-Anon with my mother. She is trying to figure out where she went wrong. How to be a better wife. In case you don't know, Al-Anon is the sister organization to Alcoholics Anonymous. Its goal is helping the families deal with the alcoholic in their lives. It's a support group of people who've been there and know the terror and frustration. The broken promises and embarrassing disappointments. They offer a sympathetic ear and encouragement to take care of yourself first, before you help someone with a drinking problem. It might be worth checking out if you haven't done so already. They are good people. The main message is the same as mine: sort yourself out – your peace isn't contingent on the approval of others.

One Al-Anon meeting when I was around eight years old, circa 1975, I went with my mother and learned about alcohol the drug. I vividly recall an old woman explaining a bit of physiology, specifically how long it would take to metabolize an ounce of alcohol. You've likely seen this chart on the written driver's license test in your state.

In any case, it takes a certain amount of time to metabolize a standard drink, depending on your biological sex and weight. I made a few calculations—I was good at math. Since my dad was drinking a quart a day of gin, it would take thirty-two hours to metabolize all the alcohol he was drinking from sunrise to sunrise. Not only was there no point in the day when he was sober, but the figures implied he was getting drunker day-by-day.

I decided right then I wasn't going to become an alcoholic. I swore to keep control should I ever drink. In doing so I was already sunk. People who have a healthy relationship with alcohol don't say things like, "I'm going to make sure it doesn't get out of hand."

I didn't know that then, but I was already on a path that would lead me here, and fortunately to survive to write this book. Later, I'll talk about the genetic aspects of chemical dependency, but in the disco era I was only a kid. Having seen firsthand what an alcoholic looked like, I didn't want to be that kind of person.

My boyhood conviction didn't sustain me, and is nonexistent by age fifteen. I am with some friends from school, about ten of us. We are at Matt's house on Friday afternoon and there are no parents around. The guys have a bottle of Southern Comfort and a case of beer. A girl I like is here, too, and I like her. I am too self-conscious to talk to her. I take a sip of the fruity, thick liquor and pass the bottle to a friend.

In a couple of minutes, I fit in a little better. I crack one of the beers. It's warm, and bitter after the syrupy So-Co, but I gulp it down. Then the most amazing thing happens: I'm not scared anymore. I confidently stride over to the object of my teen desires, and by the end of the night we are making out.

I am not afraid to talk to her. I don't mind being around other people. I feel safe and comfortable. I forget all about my Dad who is at home, fixing his own gin on the rocks. I embrace a feeling of limitless success. A magic experience, alcohol.

This powerful introduction to what chemicals can do *for* me, combined with the lack of awareness of what they are going to do *to* me becomes a strategy I deploy as often as I can. I used them with great regularity whenever I was at a party or around people and felt uncomfortable. I didn't immediately become a daily, heavy drinker, but I had a complicated relationship with alcohol from the beginning.

Booze was more than just a social lubricant. It was a way for me to let go of all these fears. It worked well, for a while. Unfortunately, the cost was very high. Instead of being uncomfortable and allowing time and genuine experience to produce a true sense of confidence, my personal identity was weakened by leaning on alcohol for support.

Because I avoided many of the challenges of adolescence (and really, forming relationships in general), my emotional development was *retarded*. I didn't know this at the time. I felt then like I had a superpower. By the time I was a teenager, things were so bad with my dad, that I was doing everything I could to be out of the house. That included more and more time with friends, and more and more time with drinking. I experimented with other substances. I didn't want the good-times to end so I took stimulants. "Bennies" or "cross-tops" or "Christmas trees." I don't remember where they came from, but they were ubiquitous and when I took them I felt strong.

In my teens years, I also tried marijuana but prefer like it as I felt groggy afterward. Nevertheless, if pot was the main course at a party, I certainly inhaled, dealing with sleepiness mañana. Partying quickly took a toll on my academic pursuits. I was far more interested in girls and "experiences" in the exiting world of 1980s Los Angeles. By tenth grade, my performance at school was so bad, the vice principal summoned me to her office to tell me I was on the verge of being expelled. Past the verge

I had an allergy to authority. When she threatens that I'm in danger of flunking out, I go to def-con one and drop out of high school. My dad weirdly supports my act of self-determination. He tells me if I'm not going to go to school, then I must get a job if I want to live at home. At fifteen, I find work delivering sandwiches to offices in the twin towers in Century City. I feel pity the office workers, trapped in their glass boxes. I patch together a few more entry-level service jobs. They give me more reason to be out of the house than they do cash money. By this point, my father isn't around much and my mother is more and more frantic that he'll leave her. Nobody seems to notice, or care, that I'm adrift.

I lean more heavily on drugs and alcohol to cope. Substances become my go-to approach for handling feelings of fear or uncertainty. Chemicals afford the option to "flee" while remaining put. I can handle the stresses of life, whether by being intoxicated or just having the quiet self-assurance that relief for my pain is around the corner. The chemical control I have over my emotions is like a subprime loan with attractive initial terms. A balloon payment is coming due. For now, though, I feel invincible despite the chaos of my family.

I decide to finish high school, partly on a dare from a girlfriend. The Vice Principal of my high school was surprised to see me. Refusing a degree-by-exam (G.E.D.), I insist on doing all the back reading and assignments for high school. I spend twelve hours a day for six months and complete the work. By the end of senior year, I am eligible to graduate with my class. Many were stunned to see me walk across the stage and receive my diploma—me most of all.

After various restaurant jobs for couple of years, I enroll at Santa Monica City College. My first class is in public speaking. I choose it because I'm both terrified to speak in front of people, and its timing fits with my work schedule. I continue to work as a waiter for rent and food money. Second semester I take a broader range of classes. Luckily I get into learning. Two more years at junior college, and I transfer to UC Berkeley to complete my undergraduate degree in molecular biology (biochemistry).

The busier I am the easier it is for me not to drink or use drugs. While I'm maximally engaged at school, I don't have a substance problem. There is no time to be stoned. I am on a mission to finish college.

Maybe my penchant for learning and academic study is itself a coping mechanism? Perhaps my quest for knowledge is a way for me to order my life and feelings. I receive accolades and approbation from my scholastic success. These are legitimate accomplishments, and pursuit of them fills up the idle time which would otherwise be spent drinking or using drugs. I wasn't aware of the mission-instead-of-drinking philosophy at the time. Looking back, however, I stumbled on a consistent truth for beating addiction: get busy. With only two years to go for my undergraduate degree. I move up Interstate 5 to the Berkeley Hills.

U.C. Berkeley is Disneyland for nerds. I've found my people. I plunge into research and the lab of Dr. Koshland. Dan is the editor of *Science* magazine. Thursdays a famous scientist visits the lab and gives us students a lunchtime talk. Many are Nobel Laureates; all are superstars and honored to visit Dr. K. After a thought-provoking discussion from this week's guest, we typically go to lunch at Dan's favorite Chinese restaurant. I'm lucky to meet many interesting people, and begin to imagine a career as an academic at a university. But I can't let go of a competing desire to be a medical doctor.

I like them both. Deciding which vision to abandon is hard. Three nights a week I volunteer at the Berkeley Free Clinic near the university. The HIV epidemic is raging, and the clinic is on the frontline of serving the homosexual, indigent, and indigent homosexual communities. People's Park swells with vagabonds. Each faces significant barriers to prompt medical care, especially for common problems like STD's or minor wounds. We provide free basic treatment and health education for anyone who presents to the clinic front desk. The clinic line stretches deep out into the parking lot.

I serve there as a lay assistant to the volunteer attending physician. I learn how to listen to patients and what to look for when formulating a diagnosis. I pick up enough medical understanding to decide my path. I choose medicine, and am fortunate enough to get into UC Davis, an hour down the road from Cal. After graduation (Linus Pauling, double-Nobel Laureate gives our commencement address), I spend the next four years split between the sleepy town of Davis, California, and the "knife and gun club" of the gang-dominated state capital.

During medical school, I hardly drink and rarely use drugs. I smoke pot only a few times during my four years. Med school is total immersion. The classic metaphor of taking in the new information in medical school is like "trying to take a drink from a firehose." I'm happier than I've ever been. I have a burning passion to learn everything. Unfortunately, I also brought with me a growing feeling of being a fraud, of the imposter syndrome.

I have the same bad dream every few nights. In it, our med school dean calls me to his office and tells me there's been a terrible mistake. How did a guy who dropped out of high school make it to *Berkeley*, and then *medical school?* This is an unshakable, guilty thought.

The factual answer is, I showed up, worked and did everything I needed to do to qualify. No one gave me anything. Good teachers certainly helped me, but I had to earn my position. A deeper part of me believed I didn't earn it. There must be some sort of mistake. Fear of expulsion haunts my whole time at UC Davis Medical School. There is a benefit to this nagging terror of being inadequate: I study my ass off.

I complete medical school but with no clear direction toward a specialty. The Department of Surgery offers me an internship. At the end of that the school year, there is an opening in the department of anesthesiology. Its Chairman offers me a residency.

One year before I began anesthesia residency, there was a federal healthcare proposal that scared nearly all doctors across the country, especially those in private practice. Government control of medicine was on the horizon and uncertainty surged. Many doctors who'd planned on retiring not only stayed on during the job, but they also had economic fears of hiring new junior associates.

This hiring freeze backed up the whole system. Many specialties were affected, and anesthesia was one of the hardest hit. Anesthesiology previously was an extremely popular specialty – good pay, early hours, decent autonomy. But the new graduates found themselves unable to get jobs, and more junior trainees left their residencies to try to switch to something else. This was a widespread panic, and it resulted in a few vacancies in training programs.

In April 1997, after having had many occasions to observe me working in the OR, Peter Moore, the department chairman, offered me a residency position. This is the first moment I've considered anesthesia as a career. He reads my surprise.

"Look, you can try it for a year and if it isn't for you, no haad feelings," Dr. Moore is from Melbourne. In his thick Australian accent, makes me an offer I can't turn down.

I start my anesthesiology residency that summer, and to my surprise, I love it. It is fun, challenging, and complex. Different cases every day, different surgeons, and different underlying medical problems. Pediatric anesthesia, cardiac, and all sorts of other things I hadn't been exposed to before, are exhilarating to participate in. The challenges are hard, fast, important. It's life and death and I don't get easily rattled under pressure. I'm good at the technical aspects of the job too. I'm also intrigued by the management of consciousness. I ponder on where we "go" when under anesthesia.

About halfway through the first year, I start to wonder about the substances we use to knock out our patients. I'm especially curious about the opiates, specifically morphine. There's nothing like countenance of bliss when morphine bathes the brain. Remembering my first drink years before, I can recall the sensation of ethanol brightening every shaded fearful corner. This sense-memory sparks a desire for the feeling again, only this time it'll be even better.

That spark of desire touched off a wildfire which nearly burned everything down. Though it was over twenty years ago, it's still hard elucidate my prior thinking. Memories lie. My recollections are refracted through the prism of intervening events. I'm doing the best I can to explain the journey from A to B. I remember at the time thinking that I just wanted to try it. I rationalized this sin, telling myself I'm a trained professional; I know what I'm doing. It takes me two months from decision to execution. I muster the "courage" to inject myself with morphine, but the two fears fought a drawn-out war.

Fear #1: I need relief that only opioids can bring, because I'm marred in some fundamental way.

Fear #2: Inject dope and I may die, but if I live I will be an I.V. drug-user.

I cadged two milligrams of the clear liquid from an opened glass vial in the emergency room. It was destined for the waste bin, but I diverted it.

When I finally inject it, the warmth eases up my arm and into my chest. Peace and calm smother my innermost thoughts. I experience the feeling of unlimited success. It is far stronger than I anticipated. I don't know if this bliss is due to the morphine, or to the insane bravado of becoming an injection drug user. Maybe both, but it is exhilarating. Some weeks pass, but I've "gotten away with it," and I steal some more morphine. On the heels of this victory, I empirically investigate the rest of the drugs used in the practice of anesthesia.

Clever as I think I am at the time, how the rules don't apply to me, I'm a garden-variety drug addict now. Within only a few months I have a habit I can't shake. The monkey is firmly attached to my scapula. Every morning, I make the same plan as the morning before: "Today is the day that I stop." By the time the workday ends, I already have more for this evening. I can't tell anybody what is happening because I'm scared of the consequences. I have the crippling habit of pure self-reliance. I've figured out most everything else on my own. I can figure out how to get out of this.

Ultimately, I can't fight alone. I need to trust another person with the truth. In the nick of time, I confess to Dr. Moore, and explain my situation. Fortunately, he is receptive and loving and kind, and he points me in a good direction: away from the hospital and toward people who trudged this path before. First steps include an indeterminate duration leave of absence from the hospital and residency program.

I martyr through detox. My only crutch for the comedown is a tub of hot bathwater. By far, these are the worst physical six days of my life. Strange thing though, psychologically they were much better than the tug-of-war every day at the hospital. Inexplicably, I knew I was done, Done, DONE. My detox felt like a rite of passage into a new life. (NB: in general, doctors dissuade people from detoxing without consulting a physician. I figured being one, I was following doctor's orders. Old habits.)

After detox, I went to three months of local A.A. meetings before shipping off to Oregon. There was a rehab facility few miles outside of Portland specializing in the treatment of doctors. Even though I'm clean and done with drugs, sober for three months, I still am forced to go to rehab.

I fought the new help, pouting that I stopped without them. Much later I learn how lucky I am. Being a physician gave me access to a program with what is still the best success rate in the addiction treatment field. It is run by State Medical Boards, and is called the Physician's Diversion Program.

Mine required a twice-a-week therapy group, frequent surprise urine testing, a demand for in-patient treatment (thus, Portland), and ongoing monitoring should I go back to work. It took three months before I could scrape together the deposit on expensive rehab. I stayed clean and was an oddity in that I didn't need detox on arrival.

I enter the program scared, entitled, arrogant, and embarrassed. By the time I graduate the Diversion Program five years later, I have a different perspective. In my three months of rehab alone, I meet nine(!) other anesthesiologists: veterans of similar journeys. My shittiest-doctor-ever self-image is cancelled. I'm a person with a problem, not a marked man. A drug or alcohol habit isn't even an uncommon problem; it's boringly common. And not just in the medical profession, but in mankind.

About one in eight people right now should probably be in addiction treatment. Over a lifetime, it's more like one in five who need to change their habits. Going through rehab reframed my understanding. The ways I thought I was bad or wrong, turned out to be the commonalities I shared with the other men and women in treatment. There was very little that was unique about my story but I didn't know that until I got sober and asked for help.

While in rehab I experimented with telling the truth. I figured I couldn't get any lower than being in rehab with a bunch of messed up doctors and lawyers. There was also one AFL union welder from New Jersey, Don, who had great health insurance. He went to rehab for a month every January.

Truth-telling was a new kind of high. If I was scared, I said so. If, for example, I heard something troubling from another rehab-mate, I told the man on the spot—not worrying if I was accurate or wrong. I stopped trying to be right and started to be honest about how I felt. It was exhilarating. My insights, drawn from my own experience, often were accurate, especially when I quit trying to be liked.

People would often bristle at my full-contact honesty, but within a day—two at most—they would usually tell me I'd nailed them with the truth. At my graduation ceremony from the rehab, the guys gifted me a fake ID badge complete with shoestring lanyard. It resembled the ones the staff wore. The picture of me was hand drawn instead of the traditional workplace mug shot, but the spirit was genuine. It had my name on it, of course. My title: Junior Counselor. Foreshadowing.

I stayed in the Diversion program for five years without relapse. I worked as a general doc-in-the-box for a two of years before Dr. Moore invited me back to complete the remaining two years of my anesthesiology residency. It was a big step and there were many people who felt my return to the OR was an unnecessary risk: for the *hospital*. In one sense, they were right to balk, but I had unfinished business. I knew I could stay sober, even back in the operating rooms.

The scorn from others was hard. I turned it into a personal challenge and was fueled to stay sober by my "colleagues" at the hospital. The long hours and low pay were familiar. But making $4 an hour after earning a good living in the urgent care clinic was tough. For my time back in residency, my wife worked as an itinerant nursing home doctor while lugging around our infant son. Let it never be said she is anything less than the best partner.

I'd already started to think about working in the field of addiction treatment. Finishing an anesthesia residency more than a small pain in the ass. Like Sir George Leigh Mallory's "because it's there" remark about Mt. Everest, I had to finish. I wasn't going to let my past ruin my future. I wanted to pay back the sacred debt to all the professors who taught me the art of medicine, as well as to my peers. Not only those who welcomed me back, but to those opposed as well. I owed them a debt too. I had disrespected the specialty and amends must be made.

Dr. Moore gave me an opportunity to change my life when he paged me. I was only a dose or two away from death. He would say he was doing his job, looking after one of his residents, but I think there were greater forces in action. Why that day? How did he know to reach out to me at the bottom of my hopeless despair? For a rational, scientist like me, the timing was more than coincidental.

He not only made it easy for me to jump off the hell-bound train, he gave me a goal to work toward as part of my recovery. In a single conversation, I went from lost to purpose-driven. He gave me hope and a goal.

To set things right at work, I had to go back and finish. To do that I had to stay sober and complete the requirements of the diversion program. My next five years were laid out, and the rubric itself was a great comfort. I knew where to go and what to do at all times. With the new habits created by all that routine, I built a sturdy frame of new habits. The new structure has stood strong since, and whenever I'm confused or uncertain, I lean on the order of routine.

I finished residency, passed my written and then oral anesthesiology boards. I worked for a year in Northern California as a cardiac anesthesiologist, but my own heart lay elsewhere. In 2005, I returned to Los Angeles, getting a job as an addiction doctor. I've been helping people just like me ever since; earning my boards in addiction medicine as well.

It has been nearly two decades since I went through the ordeal of nearly dying, fentanyl detox, and the first steps toward a new life. I haven't had a drink or a drug since. I no longer manage my feelings with chemicals.

Don't get hung up on the odd particulars of fentanyl or medicine in my tale. The backbone of my story is common. Common as ham & eggs. Society records innumerable souls who leaned too heavily on drink or drug to cope with life. Let's look in the next chapter at a few of the more interesting emotional chemists of history. You might be surprised to learn you're in good company.

☐

–7–

THE HISTORY OF ADDICTION AND TREATMENT

In 2018, President Trump declared the opioid crisis a national health emergency. The White House estimates the annual cost to be more than $500 billion, and the toll on human life is incalculable. If we include alcohol and its inevitable costs, we are over $1 trillion. Tobacco kills a half-million people a year in the US. Substance habits constitute the most expensive "lifestyle" illness in terms of financial and longevity measures.

We use a measurement called Quality Adjusted Years of Life Lost or QUALYs. Since substance habits are a developmental problem (they begin in adolescence, usually) the QUALY cost makes substance habits the number one health problem in America. Add obesity, another habit illness, and addiction commands the top step in the human misery medal ceremony. An alien visitor to Earth might wonder why we're screwing around for so long with habit-illness. Unfortunately, human beings have been dealing with this problem since we've been human beings. Maybe even before we were human.

The Mesopotamian king, Gilgamesh, threw a legendary party around 2600 B.C. He called for "ale, beer, and wine as a river, so I can give them a celebration like new year." Bangor University, Wales, is home to Dr. Mark Bellis. He's a professor of public health, and he describes the fabled king at this especially raucous celebration.

Gilgamesh was not alone among tippling rulers. Other ancients certainly knew how to drink–and boast. Alexander the Great, so the story goes, got into a drinking contest with a countryman. The man who reportedly wept because there were no more worlds to conquer made a wager. The bet:

which of them could drink an entire bowl of wine. Not a cereal bowl; a massive serving bowl–almost too heavy to lift.

Alexander "won" the bet by downing the tureen of brew. He was a badass, for sure, but he died a few days after the party. His death was likely due to acute liver failure. Obviously, drinking to death goes back beyond the mists of history. This relationship is intimately entwined with the development of civilization, and mankind itself. We see the echoes in DUI fatalities and opiate overdoses in our day.

In the U.S., public acknowledgement that excessive alcohol consumption is a national health issue begins in the late 18th century with Dr. Benjamin Rush. He was one of the signers of The Declaration of Independence. Dr. Rush founded Dickinson College in 1783. Rush University Medical College in Chicago was later named in his honor.

The doctor, in 1808, wrote a long letter to his friend, John Adams. He remarked upon the problem of people unable to stop drinking alcohol. The early American recommended, if you were a soul who struggled with temperance, you should stop completely. In his experience, Dr. Rush had yet to find anyone like this who became able to moderate his drinking.

1847, a memoir written by Luther Benson about the modern treatment of alcoholism reads as though it could have been penned in our own time. In Benson's autobiography, dramatically titled *Fifteen Years in Hell*, he recounts his own experience with alcoholism beginning with his first drink at age six. Familiar to anyone who's received an outsized effect from alcohol or drugs, he describes vividly "the warm effects" on his mind, body, and emotions. I know what he means.

He proceeds to describe a terrible period of drinking and collapse and severing of all his relationships consequently. People came to not trust him. He tried all sorts of different cures, from self-will, to religion, to joining temperance movements. Benson even became a temperance circuit speaker, and threw himself into getting other people sober. He recorded in his journal, hoping it would, as he said, "Take the place of alcohol." He writes:

"I learned too late that this was the very worst thing I could have done. I was all the time expending the very strength I so much needed for the restoration of my shattered system."

In the early 19th century people tried to manage their drinking in the same ways we do today. They cut down, or switched to beer to wine and back to beer. Countless good-sounding advice like "don't drink so much," "behave yourself," or "go to church," were as popular one hundred sixty years ago as they are today. For Luther Benson in the 19th Century, and for most drug/alcohol dependent people today, nothing worked. Benson wrote his memoir from an Indiana insane asylum. Back then it was called a home for *criminal alcoholics*.

It's not that he was a criminal; he just couldn't function in society while drinking. Being locked up was the only way to keep him away from alcohol, and it was the more humane thing to do at the time. Little has changed. There were many of these facilities in the 19th century. A huge network of them dotted New York state called Inebriety Homes. Since then, doctors, laypeople, judges, politicians, and clergy have tried all sorts of ways to sober up alcoholics. A consistent maxim is a sequester from the substance. A period of abstinence coupled with initiation of a different routine. The goal of these programs is to change the patient's perspective.

The process of revising what you think about the world, is as easy as trying to push a rope. Willingness is an indispensable ingredient for personal change. A man's opinion changed against his will is of the same opinion still. It is hard to change a point of view. Countless charlatans over centuries have offered patented "get cured quick" schemes. There is one down the road here in Malibu who'll "cure" you of your alcoholism for $90,000.

150 years ago, Leslie Keeley was a graduate of Rush Medical College and he served in the Union army as a surgeon. Following the war, he opened a practice in Dwight, Illinois, and within a few years he made a fantastic claim: "Alcoholism is a disease and I can cure it." His method resembled, in many respects, the rehabs of today. People came to the small city of Dwight, paid a significant sum of money, and lived in a therapeutic community. Hotels, boarding houses, and eventually private homes were stuffed to capacity with inebriates looking for a cure.

The cure involved a taper of whiskey over a few days followed by four-times-a-day injections of "The Keeley Gold Cure." It was a secret formula (later revealed to be 50 proof alcohol and yellow dye) promoted as "bichloride of gold" but not actually containing any gold. Cocaine might have been added at times; atropine and aloe at others. He kept the formulation a secret.

Keeley became very wealthy when he franchised the clinics in the U.S. and eventually in Europe. At the corporate zenith, there were two hundred such clinics. He died at his winter home in 1900, in Los Angeles at age sixty-three. His estate was valued at over $1 million, which would have made him one of the wealthiest men in America at the time. The clinics remained in operation, slowly shutting their doors as medical scrutiny increased. The last one closed in *1966*.

Keeley claimed people were "cured" even if they drank after treatment. He maintained, if they drank alcohol after being cured of the disease of drunkenness, it was by their own choice. Sounds like most treatment facilities today. Years later he would admit that most people relapsed. Eventually, the medical profession prevailed in outing Keeley as a quack, but that was long after he left in indelible mark on the treatment of alcoholism. In many ways, his model is still in use today.

He was a pioneer of what is now called the therapeutic community. Perhaps in part because customers/patients paid so well, he was especially kind to alcoholics. In many ways medicine is still looking for the same cure once promoted by Dr. Keeley. Doctors want to offer a treatment or medication that results in a flash of insight and a magical new life. We send people away to therapeutic communities pushed by the hope they'll sort themselves out. They are shunned for 28 days as a ritual purification and quarantine. The "demons" having fled, the addict is restored and can be safely readmitted to society. But what happens when the physician himself falls under the spell of addiction?

No historical record I can find describes Dr. Keeley as an addict, but there was another famous surgeon, William Stewart Halsted from Johns Hopkins, who fell under addiction's spell. Young Dr. Halstead, a graduate of Yale and Columbia, traveled around Europe in the late 19th century, and studied with the greatest surgeons of the Continent. In 1884, Halstead read a paper by an ophthalmologist (Köller) on the topical use of cocaine for eye surgery. Halstead's brilliant mind realized the potential of the powerful new medicine, thinking he could use it as a tool for nerve blocks. Cocaine would allow him to remove tumors and cysts without causing his patients pain. Anesthesia to this day is the greatest advance in the history surgery. Halstead advanced both fields by figuring out the anatomy of pain-nerves. He accomplished this by cocaine injection on the only study subject he had available: himself.

Anesthesiologists and surgeons still use his techniques for nerve block, though with drugs like lidocaine instead. Because of the drug's mental effect on the young surgeon, however, he became dependent on cocaine. The doctor's decline was so ghastly, that his friend, rubber magnate Harvey Firestone, had Dr. Halstead kidnapped and put on a slow boat to France. Not to cause harm to his friend, but to keep him away from coke so he could dry out. Halstead completed a painful detox over two weeks aboard the ship, but when he returned to the U.S., he picked up his old habit.

Halstead went to a Butler Mental Hospital in Providence, Rhode Island, in 1886 where they succeeded in curing his cocaine dependency – by switching him to morphine! Previous cocaine-fueled erratic behavior and rampant gossip about his addiction made Halstead unwelcome in his home state of New York. He was far calmer on morphine but the reputation was hard to shake.

Fortunately, Dr. Halstead's boss at the hospital in New York, Dr. William Osler, offered him a position at a new hospital he was building in Baltimore: Johns Hopkins. Osler knew well of his friend's problem but didn't believe it interfered with the surgeon's work. Osler, writing in his personal diary of Halstead's *morphea* use, said, "He was never able to get below three grains a day [about 200mg]." He kept up his morphine habit until he died from gallstone surgery complications at age sixty-nine, in 1922. Halstead was a very high-functioning addict.

The father of modern surgery's story goes against two fundamental sacred ideas in the current treatment of addiction. First, dependency does not always lead to incapacity. Halstead remained extremely productive until his death in old age from (ironically) surgical infection. Second, his exposure to cocaine likely set him on the path to addiction, but it wasn't the drug that caused the problem. It was the drug in Halstead. Drugs alone do not produce dependency. They take root in a person predisposed to addiction. Unfortunately, the structure of the normal human brain itself is what makes the predisposition. Under the right circumstances *anyone* can become addicted to *anything*.

Halstead switched from one substance to another. He remained a daily user of morphine for another 30 years, nonetheless mentoring a generation of the nation's surgery professors. Osler took a big risk in allowing Halsted to remain on the new Johns Hopkins staff, but he thought the greater risk for medicine would be Halstead's absence. Maybe Dr. Osler served as a surrogate conscience for Halstead–an external superego. I personally find it helps to have an ally who knows my struggles, a voice of reason in troubled times.

The rise of modernity in medicine was well underway by the early 20th century, and the rise of the efficacy of the individual was developing apace. In 1928, in England, a group formed to foster mutual spiritual support. They called themselves The Oxford Group, and their principles included an appeal to a moral authority, specifically God. As important as the almighty, they stressed the value of community. They met without a specific religion, though they were founded by Protestant minister Frank Buchman. An Oxford Group chapter consisted of small groups of people with alcohol problems, who supported one another's temperance pledges. Temperance groups go back well before the 20th century.

Fifty years earlier, in antebellum America (circa, 1845), six businessmen in Baltimore mutually pledged on their honor to abstain from alcohol. After the distinguished general of the Colonial army, they called themselves Washingtonians. By 1860, the Washingtonians numbered over half a million dues-paying members. Mutual support remained a vital element of most sobriety and recovery programs. The Washingtonian's success and national prominence, begat the Oxford group.

Bill Wilson, eventual co-founder of Alcoholics Anonymous, was introduced to The Oxford Group in the fall of 1934 by his friend and fellow New York inebriate, Ebby (Edwin) Thatcher. The five Cs of the Oxford Group – Conviction, Confession, Contrition, Conversion, and Continuance – would be expanded to the twelve steps of Alcoholics Anonymous by 1939, with the publication of "The Big Book."

Frank Buchman helped Bud Firestone, son of rubber magnate, Henry Firestone (Halstead's friend), lick his alcohol problem. Headquartered near Akron, Ohio, word of the younger Firestone's success reached Mrs. Anne Smith, the wife of a local alcoholic surgeon, Dr. Robert Smith. Smith had tried several times to stop drinking, but he relapsed repeatedly after a few weeks.

On a business prospecting trip to Akron, Wilson's hopes for a big contract fell through and, feeling sorry for himself, he looked with nostalgia at the lobby bar of the Mayflower Hotel. Wilson had been hospitalized many times with acute alcohol poisoning and he'd been told by Dr. William Silkworth, back in New York, Bill had to choose between sobriety or a painful alcoholic death.

Aware relapse might be fatal; Wilson instead went to a telephone booth and began calling the churches he found in the phone directory. Bill asked for an alcoholic to "work with," and scored a meeting in the living room of a local Akron lay-minister, and Oxford Group member, Henrietta Buckler Seiberling. She liked the young stockbroker's voice, and deciding he was sincere, arranged a meeting with the Akron proctologist and town drunk, Dr. Robert (Bob) Smith.

Seiberling's own marriage was crumbling, and she was spending considerable time with Mrs. Ann Smith, Bob's wife. Though Mrs. Seiberling's family was active in the Lutheran church, Henrietta preferred her own reading of the bible over formal church service. She reached out to her friend's husband, hoping he might help Mr. Wilson stay dry, and perhaps in the process help the surgeon get a little closer to sobriety.

Smith agreed to meet the man from New York for fifteen minutes; they talked for three hours. Smith continued to scuffle for a few more months, but their meeting planted a seed and soon after Smith quit alcohol for good. Dr. Smith stayed sober until his death in 1950. Bill returned to Brooklyn, sober, and never drank alcohol again. Henrietta Seiberling became a co-founder of the organization which would eventually be known as Alcoholics Anonymous.

The meeting between Smith & Wilson happened on June 11, 1935. Later Bill published a book with stories of the early participants, and a description of the twelve steps to become sober. For the first several years, the groups mimicked the format of an Oxford group. New Yorkers, they found, were less eager than Ohioans to embrace some of the more evangelical aspects of the Oxford groups. Alcoholics Anonymous emphasized "God, as you understand Him," a nod to more agnostic sensibilities. A.A. grew in popularity and, by the 1950s, Wilson made a pitch to The American Medical Association to reclassify alcoholism as a disease.

Reclassification of a drinking problem from moral to medical made available a new source of payment for treatment of problem drinkers: health insurance. By 1958, three-quarters of Americans were covered by health insurance. Hospitals welcomed access to insurance reimbursement, even creating special wards for drinkers drying out. Classification of addiction as a disease continues to prop open institutional checkbooks.

The re-labeling of addiction from habit to moral weakness to disease, has been a mixed bag for the heavy drinker. Revision of terminology has left the public confused as well. On the good side of the ledger, medical classification spurred research in biology and a better understanding of human behavior in general. It is also a positive result that alcoholics are less-often regarded as merely craven, but that they wrestle with a malfunctioning reward system. In point of fact, the reward system of the alcoholic is functioning just fine. It is his measurement of the value of long-term vs short-term rewards which is out of whack. Future-discounting, or failing to count the total cost, is the nemesis of the habituated. Unfortunately, neither "alcoholism is a disease," nor the NIDA's recent phrasing, "brain disease," are helpful in a practical sense. In fact, the definitions currently in vogue are counterproductive for two important reasons.

First, who among us would rather carry the label "brain diseased" over the equally unappealing "weak-willed?" Not much of a difference, if you ask me. Our medical approaches haven't been revolutionized by following the god of science instead of the ancients. Most addiction treatment facilities add a handful of psychiatric diagnostic codes to your chart (i.e., dual diagnosis) to enhance your billable profile. Health insurance companies speak the language of medical codes. More "medicalese" equals higher acuity. On average, increased acuity leads to higher profit per customer for the treating facility.

A small percentage of rehab customers are correctly classified with mental illness besides of their substance use disorder. If you think about how hard it is for a doctor to diagnose mental illness in the setting of rehab, it makes sense. The typical rehab customer bounces all over the place emotionally.

When a person has a substance habit, his psychological responses are, obviously, under the influence of that substance. During detox, he's in withdrawal and displays a different spectrum of symptoms and responses. Soon after detox, the lack of routine previously enforced by the habit cycle of using, causes a new type of psychological stress and a different presenting picture to the clinicians with the clipboards. It's tough out there for a shrink.

Depending on when a customer is interviewed by the mental health professionals, he may get tagged with a mood disorder diagnosis (e.g. bipolar), a thought disorder (such as paranoia from marijuana use, or DTs from alcohol withdrawal) or literally anything in the latest edition of the psychiatric diagnosis manual (DSM).

Another reason it is hard to grow up and change your substance habits is practiced helplessness. Refusal to accept personal responsibility for your own actions is a crippling habit. In many ways, defining substance habits as a "brain disease" is the 21st century way of saying "the devil made me do it." If imbalanced chemicals in your brain are responsible for your ongoing substance habits, regardless of the clear damage to you and those around you, then you can keep partying without guilt. You're just warped that way; so, bottom's up. The following story will illustrate why the concept of "brain disease" can't possibly be the whole story.

American troop withdrawal during "Vietnamization" of the Vietnam War, coincided with the start of Richard Nixon's second term as President. He was worried the demobilization of three hundred thousand battle-hardened, drug-addicted G.I.s returning stateside would be in another withdrawal: this one from ubiquitous Vietnam heroin.

Up to one-quarter of them became addicted to heroin while fighting in the jungles. Sure, a few had prior chemical addiction before shipping out. But most of the soldiers who smoked or injected themselves with the readily available opiates did so to deal with the terror of war itself. With all those addicted soldiers repatriating, President Nixon proclaimed, "America's public enemy number one in the United States is drug abuse. In order to fight and defeat this enemy, it is necessary to wage a new, all-out offensive."

Our second-wave prohibition followed a similar philosophy to that employed a half-century earlier. The Nixon administration policy was to cut off the supply of drugs. How else to solve the problem of addiction? Interdiction of transport, and pursuit of the dealer's network, was the standard playbook. This required a large law enforcement contingent. The Drug Enforcement Agency (DEA) focused on the "French Connection," heroin manufacture in Vietnam.

Popular conception said heroin addicts were beyond help. The substance turned them in to single-minded ravenous beasts, or so people feared. We had to bring our boys home, but the question of how to do so safely vexed our leaders.

Alcoholics Anonymous was flourishing in the 1970s, claiming an active membership of around two million, but their community was closed to people addicted to drugs. In my own hometown, we had a notorious treatment center for drug addicts called Synanon. Their headquarters were located in the same structure that today is the beautiful Hotel Casa del Mar in Santa Monica, California.

Synanon, was founded in 1958 by Charles Dederich, a former member of Alcoholics Anonymous who had a drug problem. A charismatic speaker, he was still shushed by AA members because Dederich insisted on talking about his personal use of drugs, especially heroin. Though it eventually was exposed as a brainwashing cult, Synanon had some success helping heroin addicts kick the habit. This caught the attention of President Nixon and he considered the Synanon program for the returning Vietnam vets.

Theirs was a community support model, but enhanced with peer confrontation of "negative behavior." In practice, it entailed screaming profanities and insults at their members in order to "break them down." This was allegedly done for their own good, and with the hope Synanon clients would put themselves back together sober. Complete obedience to Dederich was required.

Ascetic self-denial as a pathway to enlightenment is an ancient method, but we better be suspicious when the rehab guru demands you give over your worldly possessions to him as a condition of salvation. Through aggressive litigation, Synanon fended off the authorities for two decades. Eventually the Internal Revenue Service retroactively withdrew their tax-exempt status as a non-profit.

Dederich expanded its ministry to "squares," those without a substance problem but who sought enlightenment. Synanon was thriving, and owned $33 million worth of California real estate, ten airplanes and 400 vehicles. Non-profits could be very profitable. This caught the attention of law enforcement and an investigation of abuse, rape and torture rumors followed.

Two Synanon "Imperial Marines," Lance Kenton and Joe Musico, severed the rattle from a diamondback rattlesnake (so it gave no audible warning) and hid it in the mailbox of Los Angeles District Attorney Paul Morantz. The D.A. was bitten by the serpent; a neighbor applied a tourniquet. Synanon did not survive.

The pioneering rehab, once heralded as a beacon for returning Vietnam vets, was exposed as rotten with corruption. Dederich and Musico were found guilty of attempted murder and incarcerated.

Unfortunately, this is a recurring archetype in addiction treatment. A larger-than-life personality anoints himself the fount of health and recovery, as we've seen with Keeley, Buchman and Dederich. In this style of rehab, you must obey. If you object to any part of the treatment paradigm, that's your disease talking. Snake-oil salesmen and charlatans have been with us always, but it's distressingly common here in Malibu to hear someone say they have a "cure" but only if you check in immediately to their facility. Oh yeah, better bring fat stacks of cash.

There are also myriad treatments in the medical world claiming to restore chemical balance that we mentioned earlier. They include vaccines aimed at the immune system inducing it to attack substances (drugs) if they come into the body. Other treatments include chemicals to block receptors, so that when you take the drug it has no effect. These medicines either block the effect of opioids (naltrexone), or they make you sick by blocking an intermediate enzyme step (disulfiram). Still others are meant to adjust your mood and thoughts (antidepressants). So far, they have been at best blunt instruments; more hammer than scalpel. This vector of approach sounds scientific, but there is one stubborn problem: the brain is smarter than the drugs we give it. How do we know this? Tolerance.

The brain adapts, given time, to all drugs. It accommodates the effect of a substance by reducing the sensitivity of each neuron. This accounts for tolerance and, when you stop taking a drug, withdrawal symptoms. Why would we think the brain doesn't develop tolerance to *any* drug that affects brain function? It's built to adapt and deal with the presence of any persistent substance.

I support the use of targeted psychiatric treatment in order to help people who suffer from both chemical use disorder and mental illness, (e.g. depression or bipolar). Psychiatrists can be very helpful in the small percentage of people who suffer from both. Sadly, the term "dual diagnosis" is stretched beyond recognition in many rehab facilities. A psychiatric diagnosis can be oddly seductive to those who don't want to abstain from drugs and alcohol—an alibi of sorts. Some nurture the notion it is really depression, or maybe an attachment disorder, that lies at the bottom of their struggles.

If someone is merely temporarily down, maybe an antidepressant prescription might be able to restore their constitution that of a normal drinker. "Self-medicating" was the watchword in the '90s. Although that phrase has fallen out of favor, it's much of the foundation to justify medication prescribing practices by many addictionologists. It provides cover for drinking and using by the patients. In other words, they're not drinking because they *want to*. With every substance habit treatment concept, we must be honest about the yield. In some cases, with a lifted depression (for example) casual substance use, the occasional drink of alcohol, may again be possible.

This can happen, but it's uncommon. At the heart of a substance habit, there is an issue with the way the person sees himself, especially his relationship to others. As a consequence, if he uses drugs or alcohol to deal with feelings of inadequacy, the same disappointing results will occur; he'll probably never repair his relationships. In other words, if you think you're "broken" and only a drink (drug) will fix you, then you'll never get better. One of the hardest things to do at my job is to convince a person he's okay.

These negative beliefs do worsen real psychiatric problems, and the psychiatric issues can exacerbate the fractured sense of self and prompt further substance use. A vicious cycle. Though addiction/habit worsens psychiatric illness and vice-versa, they are separate problems. One does not explain the other. If they're both present, they should both be treated.

The passé model of the "self-medication" hypothesis, is summarized: people without access to proper psychiatric diagnosis and treatment (meds) make do with whatever psychoactive chemicals they can find. It purports that attention-deficient people will use stimulants, while the anxious will drink or use sedatives. You get the idea. Though logical-sounding premise, it has failed to be the Rosetta Stone of addiction diagnosis, let alone treatment. The self-medication hypothesis is the forerunner of the buzz phrase "chemical imbalance." We can do better.

Don't surrender either your personal responsibility for sobriety or your obligation for your own mental health. Sobriety improves mental health and appropriate treatment of mental illness makes sobriety better. Each is necessary, but neither on its own is sufficient.

☐

-8-

NEUROSCIENCE OF ADDICTION AND TREATMENT

In 1954, Peter Milner and Abraham Olds published a scientific paper on electrocuted rat brains which changed the field of addiction. The two graduate students described the behavior of their furry subjects; each rat had an electrode carefully implanted into a central part of its brain called the nucleus accumbens.

The rats were placed, individually, into a "Skinner Box" (a cage designed by B.F. Skinner to record rat responses), so each animal's behavior could be studied. When the rat pressed a lever, it got a tiny little electric shock deep into a very specific part of the brain. Don't think of the experimental setup like an electric chair. It's more like when you go to the audiologist and listen for the faintest tone to test your sense of hearing. Only instead of an audio beep through the headphones, a wire is surgically placed directly into your brain.

Don't worry about the test procedure causing the little rodent any pain. The shock isn't a jolt to the rat. Similar to the tingling sensation you feel in your pinky when you bang your elbow at the "funny bone," the stimulus produces a phantom feeling *as if* that circuit of the brain were activated. When you bang your elbow just right, you feel the tingle far away from the blow: in your little finger. It's "funny" that a bang here makes tingles way over there in the hand.

The rat (or human) brain has no pain receptors. It cannot distinguish the tiny electrical stimulation Milner & Olds rigged up, from the same part of the brain being activated the normal way. Depending on where the tip of the electrode is placed, the tiny micro shock could produce all sorts of sensations or actions. A flick of the rat's tail, a tap of its clawed foot, vomiting, or in Milner & Old's precise experimental placement, the pleasure equivalent as if our little rat just snorted a fat line of cocaine.

Remember, no actual drugs are involved. The electrical pathway stimulated by the implanted electrode is the same circuit involved in the dopamine pleasure cascade. Cocaine releases a flood of dopamine in the nucleus accumbens, and the scientists figured out how to hack that pathway. At least in rats. Like the little-finger tingling, the sensation of cocaine was mimicked by the microzap. As far as the rats were concerned, they were in a bathroom stall, at Studio 54, in 1978. The coolest part: the rats could press a lever as much as they wanted to. The more they did, the more they probably felt like they Tony Montana in *Scarface*.

The rats with an electrode deep in this area of the brain pressed the lever to get another tingle down the wire. They would press and press, just for the chance to get another tiny zap. They skipped dinner and drinks (food pellets & water). Both of which also release dopamine in the same part of the brain, but food & water are much weaker stimuli for the feeling of pleasure than the electrode's bolt. Instead, they ceaselessly pressed, smacked and stomped on the lever of pleasure.

The electric-cocaine rats eventually starve to death, poor dears. Every rat brain was autopsied and carefully examined. The brain was altered beyond simply the presence of the microelectrode. The experiment revealed the neural mechanism of a habit loop; predictable control of the internal state of mind. Under the microscope the rat reward centers were damaged, literally excited to death. These findings also implied why it can be so hard to stop a habit.

Not all rats showed the same response to the electric tingles. Some rats jumped on the lever a lot, then inexplicably quit abruptly. Despite the easy comfort offered by pressing the switch, this population wouldn't touch the lever again after (perhaps) swearing off. These rats displayed true avoidance, even after the lever was reprogrammed to deliver a food pellet through a tiny door. These "abstinent" rats also had their brains examined afterward. Parts of neural tissue away from the nucleus accumbens viewed under a microscope resembled the brain of a terrified rat. Their fear centers (amygdala) were stuck in the "on" position. Perhaps trauma left lasting effects (bad trip?) and they associated the lever press with danger.

Alternate locations of electrode implantation, when stimulated, produced no visible effect. Like neurological Lewis & Clark, an early pleasure map of the rat brain was charted.

Only in this case, Olds and Milner found the mythical northwest passage: the pathway of pleasure. Pressing the lever and getting that sensation of triggering the nucleus accumbens became the model researchers used to explain addiction. Right here is where I believe the concept of "brain disease" was born. Addictive behavior is a stimulation loop that keeps itself going. Like Willard in the Skinner box, we're basically bigger rats. Only we call the dealer, hit the dispensary, or slap money down on the bar and order a stiff one. Habit.

Why evolution favored the reward and punishment feedback loops was not the focus of their study. Although all animals have some version of the pleasure circuit, the implications of this ubiquity remain underappreciated. Researchers emphasize the pathology of this system. Clinicians like me are focused on restoring normal function to the brain's awareness/decision/action system. But what if the brain of the addict isn't broken?

Trillions are spent trying to coax the brain to act right relative to others in society. Looked at for behavioral and habit control, you could make the case government itself is instituted among men in order to restrain our baser habits and foster the beneficial ones. Even more profound, it seems all creatures seek and enjoy mind-altering substances. If every creature uses mind altering chemicals as it can find them, indeed merely stimulating the same part of the brain in rats as in humans we can "create" addicts, we must consider the formation of habit loops as a *feature* of evolution, not a bug. Put simply, a habit taken to addiction may not always be bad for a species.

There is another area near the nucleus accumbens neighborhood of the brain called the ventral tegmental area, or VTA. When stimulated, the VTA also produces similar results that Olds and Milner found in the zapped rat study. Further research revealed the VTA releases a molecule called dopamine. Dopamine's role in human behavior is so central, venture investor Shawn Parker recently admitted Facebook engineers built the social media platform with the user's dopamine cascade in mind.

Combine two findings, rats isolated in boxes will press levers forever, and dopamine is in the VTA, and you've got yourself the "dopamine hypothesis" of addiction. Stated as "addiction is a malfunction in the handling of the neurotransmitter dopamine." This bolsters the "addiction = brain disease" concept, but it sheds no new light. We like simple, mechanistic explanations. Brain broke, is really simple; who cares if it's wrong, right? Pat answers are always insufficient to explain the complexities of the human mind. That doesn't stop people from tossing them around.

In 1990, Blum, et. al, published a paper in the respected *Journal of the American Medical Association* titled "Allelic Association of Human Dopamine D2 Receptor Gene in Alcoholism." Sounds like a eureka moment, no? Dr. Blum seems to be saying alcoholism = dopamine problem. Let's look more closely.

Blum looked at two structural versions of a cell-surface protein found in all humans: the dopamine receptor. He had brain samples from a few dozen cadavers diagnosed (in life) as alcoholic. Another few dozen brain samples he reported were from "normal" or non-alcoholic people.

He concluded the teetotalers were more likely to have the D1 form, and the boozers more often sported the D2 version. Attempts to repeat Blum's research have been unsuccessful. By the following year, dozens of research papers from other laboratories reported minimal or no linkage between D2 and alcohol use disorder. Unfortunately, the mechanistic idea stuck and "chemical imbalance" is thrown around as if there were solid science to back it up. Remember, we like simple. Blum's idea is incredibly persistent and still drives alcoholism research and policy. Humans like to have someone or something to blame, especially if the concept is understandable. We hate uncertainty so much, we will listen to anyone with perceived authority on a subject.

Recruiting Grammy-winning musician, Macklemore (Benjamin

Haggerty), for his March 16, 2016, Oval Office address, Barak Obama discussed the concept of addiction-as-disease. Both men related their own struggles with the habit-forming cycle of substances. Macklemore was invited an advocate of compassionate help for those caught in a substance habit. The President, a self-reported former drug user (see: choom gang), says he left smoking (marijuana) behind. Though Obama admitted each addict is different, and "genes may be a factor," he emphasized the lack of choice as a hallmark of addiction. Here the Commander-in-Chief and I part company. Specific choices may not make sense to someone watching the addict's behavior, but in the mind of the user, continued use makes sense.

Let's go back to the brain model for a moment. The nucleus accumbens (NAc) and ventral tegmental area (VTA) are hailed as the location of addiction in the brain. Blum's that dopamine hypothesis is debunked. Scientists have learned buckets more since Olds and Milner's 1954 paper too.

We now have the tools of functional MRI machines and optogenetics. fMRI is just like a regular imaging scan of the brain but overlaid with markers of brain activity. Using functional MRI (fMRI), we can see which parts of the brain are active during certain activities. Optogenetics, controlling DNA with light, allows researchers to change the activity of genes in living animals. With this impossible-to-believe technique, light-sensitive genes are inserted into "start" areas of DNA.

With a beam of light shined directly on the brain of a genetically modified *living* animal, individual genes can be switched on or off. Studies on the "reward centers" revealed dopamine surges with rewards and punishments (aversive stimuli). Turns out, dopamine isn't a marker of reward at all, but instead it signals relevancy (salience) of an event. Food and sex spike dopamine, but so do loud noises and pain. Dopamine spikes in the brain say, "Look here! This is important!" Shawn Parker was on to something, but let's lay to rest the vaunted dopamine hypothesis. Dopamine doesn't indicate a reward for pleasure, but a flag stuck on anything important.

Some of the most exciting research today is conducted by Texas A&M University researcher Brian Anderson. The professor has an idea that makes sense to me. He says addicts are not any different from ordinary people. We are all the same. The habituated have the same neural architecture as the un-addicted. Addicts and non-addicts carry out the same brain functions identically, and they react in the same way to salient stimuli. "Normal people" avoid pain and seek pleasure–same as addicts and alcoholics.

We have the same genes too. Remember the "drugs hijack the brain" concept? It holds the neurons in the brain can't distinguish between its own neurotransmitters and drugs ingested. The interplay between the built-in *this matters* (saliency) circuits, and the effects of a drug, distort and bend the judgments made the affected brain. Another important conclusion from this vantage is anyone can become an addict. Genes are neither curse, nor salvation where habit development is concerned.

Anyone, by this theory, can be turned into an addict. Everyone can, through repeated action (habit) redefine what's important. Ten years ago, there almost were no smartphones, now practically everyone has one–and we check them every five minutes! Even touching them makes us feel better, and for many, it's their first action of the day. This implies we don't even need a drug to develop a choice-control loop problem. Any behavior can become like second nature.

Professor Anderson trains people via a stimulus associated with something addictive (say, a picture of a syringe, or a meth pipe), and a parallel stimulus crafted to distract them at the same time (maybe a photo of some house keys, or a bicycle). It's kind of like Ivan Pavlov with the dogs. If you don't know about Pavlov, the story goes that he rang a bell while his dogs were eating. The dogs got so used to the sound of the bell when they were chowing down, that Ivan could ring the bell and they would begin to salivate in anticipation of dinner, before they saw any food. So, it was this other sound, the bell ringing, which prompted the pooches to salivate, and no longer the food per se.

Dr. Anderson set up his study subjects with a clever test system. He showed on a screen, drug images alternating with these irrelevant (distracting) pictures to both former addicts and non-addicts. As he showed his subjects the pictures, their brain function was tracked in a sophisticated fMRI scanner. The brains of both addicts and non-addicts adapted to seeing the competing stimuli. Repeat firing of neurons in the brain developed a habit.

Awareness was a given, since the images filled the participants' view screen. After hundreds of images, the volunteer's brains were trained to regard associated stimuli (triggers) as attention-worthy. This process happened whether the subject was an addict or not. They became "hooked" and responded to non-drug images simply because they paid attention to them. They developed a habit of liking a photo of car keys.

That to which we pay attention is important (salient). Dr. Anderson uncovered the systems that determine choice–systems integral to every human brain. He showed they function *normally* in addicts. So much for the "brain disease." The brains of addicts are indistinguishable from non-addicts in the only way that matters: the formation of habit.

We label as 'good' right now, substances and behaviors which we know are destructive in the long term. Not only are we in the habit of using the drug or taking a particular action, but we are in the habit of assigning value as well. The simplest way to predict the future is do the same thing over and over until you crave it. Addiction is more of a habit than we want to admit.

There's another interesting result from a study by Barry and Marshall at Yale and Brown, respectively. They focused on war veterans with opioid-treated chronic pain and their tendency of switching to heroin. Surprisingly, they only found an increased likelihood of heroin use in chronically opiate-prescribed vets who had a *prior narcotic abuse history.*

In other words, most of our vets take their pain medication as prescribed and don't misuse it, rarely do they go on to become heroin addicts. This is an important study. Usually we hear reports in the news like "heroin users began with opioid painkillers" but this is the wrong way to look at it. Most people who take opioids as prescribed don't progress to addiction. When I was in medical school, the number discussed was around 1 percent. It's probably a bit higher, maybe double that, but not much more. We don't really know, but the incidence is low. In the absence of prior substance abuse history, opioids used correctly rarely progress to addiction. This is true even in poor veterans with depression and/or PTSD. Takeaway: it isn't the drug that makes the addict, it's the habit.

The vets' economic status, PTSD, social support and so forth, were not nearly as influential as having a prior history of abusing pain medicine. Why do I mention this? Because when you're used to a certain coping strategy for dealing with discomfort or pain, the strategy becomes automatic. It solidifies into one that you deploy automatically. Without thinking. Pavlov's dogs? They were not thinking about salivating when they heard the bell. The pups associated a previously irrelevant stimulus with suppertime. Makes me wonder how many relapses were precipitated by irrelevant stimuli. Remember Bill Wilson, founder of AA's story in the hotel lobby bar? The sounds of conversation and piano music almost did him in.

Humans with a craving for a substance don't conceptualize the craving itself, they just feel an urge to use the drug. Prior to desire for the substance, a feeling touches off the craving. A motivation for a new state triggers the urge for action, the object of the action is a new feeling (i.e. less pain). I agree with Dr. Brian Anderson's proposition that desire for emotional control explains a lot about drug relapse. Associative cues remind us to miss the feeling of escape the drug or drink provides.

A story will illustrate what I'm talking about. The other day a former patient of mine, a young woman who's triumphed over her heroin habit going on two years, texted me about a close call. She'd gone to visit an old friend, as he asked for her help and support in his effort to get clean himself. Shocked when she got to his home, her friend was cooking up a dose of heroin in a spoon. He wrapped a tourniquet around his own arm, and hunted a vein to pierce.

She turned her back so as to not see him shoot up. Freaked out, she fled back to her apartment in the city. For several days, she fought using heroin again. When the struggle was too much, she picked up the telephone and asked for help. She didn't relapse, but it was a close call. The visual and other sensory cues almost took her down. In A.A. there is a saying about staying out of bars and other places where intoxication is the point. I've heard, "if you hang around the barbershop long enough, you're going to get a haircut."

Neural architecture, the way our nerve cells connect to each other, correlates with brain function. Most information coming our way is irrelevant to our individual survival; watch the evening news if you're not yet convinced. Over millions of years our mammalian progenitors evolved specialized neural circuits to rapidly detect important patterns. Some detection circuits are more sensitive than others. Humans have outstanding color vision. We're especially sensitive around 540nm (green) on the visible light spectrum.

We can see thousands of subtle shades of spring, lime, Kelley and olive green because our tree-dwelling ancestors were more likely to survive if they could spot the snake amongst the leaves. We categorize most information into four bins: Can I eat it? Can it eat me? Can I have sex with it? Fourthly, the biggest bin of all: Is it irrelevant background?

Daniel Kahneman in his book, Thinking Fast and Slow, gives a wonderful summary of the paleo-brain (ancient brain) that accomplishes primary threat/opportunity decision making, far below the level of conscious thought. He calls it System One, and it's essentially automatic. No wonder it is so hard to stop seeing the drink or drug as immediate relief. No wonder once we're in the grip of a habit it's so hard to stop.

Over millions of years our mammalian progenitors perfected habit systems at a level far beneath conscious thought. The way our brains categorize information determines if it is opportune, dangerous, or just background noise. Our attention determines what is salient and relevant. Let me say that again. If we don't focus on it, it may as well not exist. Dopamine spikes correlate with the salient, not the pleasurable. We breathe without thinking, though we can for a minute or two consciously hold our breath. Most of the time, the functioning brain is on autopilot, guiding our actions.

The unknown includes the opportune, the deadly and the meh. Our sorting device, the magnificent brain, is beautifully crafted to save energy. It will wire an automatic circuit to spare precious conscious attention, whenever it can. Our brains are evolved to repeat the pleasurable not only because it feels good, but by doing so we reduce shrink the territory of the unknown. If addiction is a disease, then everyone has it.

So that's the underlying history and architecture of addiction. It's not an illness that comes from outside of an individual. It isn't something we're exposed to as a virus or induced as a byproduct of a drug. We may pick up useful, resilient habits from our family or community; we can pick up bad habits too. We may also be a little more (or less) susceptible to genetic influences, but genes are not the *reason* anyone drinks his life away. We are all built to process threats and opportunities so rapidly that we don't give a second thought to the accuracy of our emotional, intuitive, ancient brains.

The point is that attention biases, things that grab the mind, are not fully within our own control. Much of our responses to the world are instinctual. We have to make a deliberate effort in order to change the things we focus upon. It's a constant effort to steer away from self-destructive habits, at least until the new, health habit is formed.

My favorite metaphor of habit-effort to illustrate recovery from an ongoing addiction problem is the image of a man climbing up the stairs of a "down escalator." If you just stay on your same tread, it's going to eventually deposit you on the floor below.

You have to keep walking in order to just stay in place. You have to hustle if you want to go up. More effort is required. The brain, trying to seek pleasure and trying to avoid discomfort, will naturally drift toward those kinds of rewards that serve its expedient purpose: get out of discomfort/minimize uncertainty. It is just trying to protect you. The "disease" does not want you dead, despite what you might hear in a 12-step meeting. Your brain is trying to keep you safe, fed, and reproductive. Fighting the brain is exhausting, but redirecting it is very useful. Habit loops are built to last.

This explains why getting sober is so hard. It also explains why relapse to old substance behaviors often yields humiliating results. Reactivate a habit, especially one which once made you feel very good, and you'll go right back to where you left off. The neural architecture you built over years is intact. The hardest habits to kick are those which make you feel in control. The brain remembers the good times and the predictability of being in the habit cycle. It's like a rip tide tugging you back out to sea. The energy efficient brain automates an anti-discomfort circuit; the tide is within. This is why we might want to be compassionate to our brothers and sisters who struggle wit substance habits. We do better with external support to change embedded habits.

Habit change is so much easier when we can contextualize our actions: some extra cues, other ways of seeing pattern, recognizing the stimulus at its inception. It's practically impossible to fight urges or cravings along with the brain that created the self-destructive/pain-avoiding circuit. Trying to do so pits us against the most successful system for survival and comfort-seeking that evolution has produced. However, if we bring these processes of threat-detection and relief-seeking up to the level of consciousness, we have a better chance to change.

If we pay conscious attention to our habits— raise awareness up to our analytic mind rather than automatic loops— then we can use our innate power for good. Paying careful attention to our actions, largely the province of the prefrontal cortex, is the best way to shelve old habits of addiction. Replacing old habits, we no longer want with preferred new ones is key too. That's where the latest neuroscience theories are directed: reframing attention.

To conclude our discussion of neuroscience and treatment of addiction, let's turn to Dr. Bruce Alexander's famous experiment from the 1970s: Rat Park. Remember when we started the chapter talking about rats with needles in their brains, getting tiny zaps of electric current? Milner & Olds's experiment is rooted in the behavioral conditioning world of legendary behaviorist B.F. Skinner. Let's look a little more closely at Dr. Skinner's experiments.

The concept is best summarized in the architecture itself of the so-called "Skinner Box." The Harvard professor designed an experimental setup consisting of an enclosure (cage), a response lever that delivers a reward or punishment (i.e. food pellet) and that allows controlled stimuli to be administered to the animal and its responses observed. In Skinner's original experiments he used a rat, but the principle can be (roughly) applied to humans as well. It's interesting to note, at one point during WWII, Dr. Skinner ran an army program that taught pigeons how to steer a missile. The development of RADAR ended his project, but he along the way he taught them to play ping pong. Look it up.

The accepted model of addiction in the brain is simply conditioned behavior following reward. The rat presses the lever, and it gets a reward. The "pleasure" stimulus in various experiments ranged from a little pellet of food that dropped when the rat pressed the lever, to others wherein the rat got a drop of alcohol or squirt of morphine into its jugular vein. Millner, you'll recall, used a few microvolts of electricity directly in the rat brain, producing the same observed effect as if it had received morphine.

Dr. Bruce Alexander, up in Canada at Simon Frasier University, and his graduate students rethought the most basic addiction model itself. They considered how the rats in these experiments are treated compared with how rats live in the wild. They're usually kept alone in a single small steel cage; one rat per box. Researchers don't want the rats tangling up their IV, catheters, or pulling their wires out by tussling with other rats. Scientists want to determine direct behavioral correlation between reward and behavior. You also won't believe what mischief a pair of rats will get up to.

Two rats or more per cage and there would be no way to know which pressed the lever or got the pellet of food. They're trapped in this small space, and they've got their lever, and they've got some water, and they have their drug that comes from the lever-pressing (or a brain zap). The intent is to collect enough data on enough rats so that you can make some statistical sense out of what they're doing. From the rat findings, we make national drug policy.

But if you saw a bank of rat cages, you would immediately notice a cage is not the natural environment for a rat. The rats are isolated in tiny rooms. Real estate in a research lab is costly so they're packed tighter than a Tokyo subway car during the commute into the city. Rats are social animals; without other rats to mingle with and conduct their ratty business, the rodents probably feel sad and scared. I would. An alternate plausible explanation for why the rats so eagerly smacked the morphine lever is they're freaked out living like a, well, like a rat in a cage.

Dr. Alexander and his team took the clever step of building an environment that more closely matched what rats actually do and how they live. They built what came to be known as Rat Park. By cage standards, Rat Park was a very large area. It was a couple of table tops, and for the rats, this was a lot more like what they were used to. They could run, they could go to different areas, there were places for them to hide and hang out with each other and sleep, and there was even an exercise wheel. The rats could also "cuddle" with their opposite gendered rats and do what came natural, if they felt amorous. Dr. Alexander provided his test subjects with two sources of hydration. One was plain water, and the other was a solution of morphine and water. According to the "hijacker" theory of "addictive substances," the rats should have all been wasted on morphine soon after they checked into Rat Park.

Surprisingly, the rats in the experimental park had no interest in water laced with morphine. They went through a number of iterations on the experiment, trying to see if they could convince the rats to prefer the morphine water. Morphine is bitter, so they added sweetener to it. Rats love sweet, but they hate bitter more. In Rat Park, they were not interested at all in the morphinated water.

Even when the amount of sugar was jacked up to maple syrup levels, the rats were not interested in morphine drinks. They even tried taking some of the rats that had become forcibly addicted them to morphine in a Skinner Box, (think Sinatra in the classic scene from *Man with the Golden Arm*) and moved them from their cages to Rat Park. These were dopesick rats; they were coming off high morphine doses and kicking hard. Alexander put them in Rat Park, with a big bottle of morphine-water right in front of them. All they had to do was skitter over and take a few pulls on the nozzle, and their pain would stop. But no. The other rats comforted them and they followed Nancy Reagan's pithy advice. In a few days, they were just another rat in the race. They quit a class A morphine habit without spending a day in rehab or a minute in a therapist's chair.

Alexander published his study. Though the grad students at Simon Frasier were impressed, in the broader addiction community the results of Rat Park were unwelcome. The mechanistic behavioral model, of rats pressing levers, was much easier to understand than the question raised by Alexander's experiment: What is addiction?

Why is it when people (or rats) are isolated, they act a certain way? When they're in a social environment, they behave completely differently. Maybe our understanding is inadequate, and maybe the way we're treating people shouldn't be like putting them in a cage like a rat. Yes, I'm talking about the prison system. Rehab too. Should we shut down all the rehabs and welcome the addicts back into their families and communities?

The rat park experiment has been repeated, but the results were not as clear as the first study. Funding was withdrawn and Dr. Alexander was encouraged to stop his research along this line of inquiry. Are these rats close enough in their drug responses to human beings? Do people just need to be around other people in a supportive, normal environment until drugs become progressively less interesting? We don't know for sure, but I think so. Doctor Alexander brushed up against the social context of saliency. What matters most depends on who you're with. Is it just me, or is that obvious?

When I see people make an attempt to get sober, they usually hang out with other people doing the same thing. This is quite frequently around the recovery community, but not always. It works commonly also via a person's religious affiliation. Remember, the Washingtonians were just businessmen in Baltimore who pledged to support each other. Geography and similar work histories were enough glue to form a common bond betwixt them. They created supportive communities and made their own Rat Parks.

People who become part of a mutual support group if they stick with it, will eventually get traction and move forward. They nearly always improve the quality of their life. I'm a pragmatist about which groups. Personally, I love AA, but anything that helps you change from habits you don't want to ones you do is fine by me.

Maybe just as important as getting better, those who join a supportive community develop a network, a system, for staying off of the substances.

Much of our empathetic connections to other people, neurologically, are centered in a group of brain cells called "mirror neurons." When you see someone receive a blow or sustain an injury, the sympathetic pain you feel is connected to a part of your brain that feels vicariously. Heck, you don't even have to see it; just hearing about something painful will do the trick. The other day at dinner, my wife's father was telling a story about leaning his palm against a hot pizza oven. As he told us that detail, we all felt the searing pain.

The scientific work on mirror neurons and empathy (oxytocin?) is yet to be fleshed out, but I think sharing our struggles and aspirations with others about quitting drugs and alcohol, is the most efficient path to beating addiction. We need partners in the journey of life; nobody succeeds alone.

We literally connect with additional minds, and their perspectives of our behavior (as well as their modeling) serve as additional data we can use to make our own better decisions. Feeling better without the drink/drug becomes another salient experience upon which we can build a new habit.

Collect enough of these warm-fuzzies and you develop a competing salience impression that steers you away from the substances. This also explains why relapse is so common. The association patterns are all still there, ready to be reactivated on short notice. You have to build a system that recognizes different patterns, such as "sobriety is key for me to reach my goals" or, "alcohol leads to pain." Unless your life improves sober, you're going to go back to using. Doctor's advice: make your own Rat Park.

–9–
WHAT TO DO IF YOU HAVE A PROBLEM

At this point you might be thinking, Cool stories doc. But what do I do about *my* problem with drinking/drugs? This is what we've been working toward. I've told you how I got here, and how I became an addiction doctor. You also know the historical threads that lead to our current treatment approaches. We have also looked at addiction from a neuroscience standpoint and learned why it isn't fair to call it a disease. In the 21ˢᵗ century, we can do a lot about habits, especially substance dependence. Let's dive in.

Since nobody does anything without checking Google first, chances are, you've looked around for help on the Internet. You've, no doubt, come across a number of websites that have urged you to talk to one of their intake coordinators or to "Call now to speak with a counselor." The treatment industry has its own lingo to describe the various intensity levels of care offered. Hospitalization, residential intensive, residential, intensive outpatient, medication-assisted therapy, counseling, and other subsets of treatment are hard for the customer to understand. In addition, there are thousands of therapists and counselors in independent practice who offer addiction treatment services.

Beyond state licensees (including chiropractors, acupuncturists, heck, maybe even manicurists), there are scads of people who trumpet their prowess in curing addiction. Chakra-balancers, shamen and shawomen of all tribes, reiki healers, séance guides, and fortune tellers all offer their services to help you obtain happiness and freedom from addiction. There are still more thousands of psychiatrists and general doctors who prescribe medications in an effort to be helpful guides to a better way of living.

There are over one hundred methadone clinics just in California. The U.S. has over fifteen thousand treatment centers. On a day like today, according to SAMHSA, the government arm of substance abuse treatment advocacy, there are over a million Americans in some form of treatment. Unfortunately, since there is no clear understanding of exactly what addiction is (disease, habit, etc.), it naturally follows that the treatment plans for addiction are a jumble too. Something isn't working and we've known this inconvenient truth for decades. Most stakeholders in the treatment industry advocate for expanded access to their version of treatment. In a subsequent chapter, we will look at their efficacy rates, and you can decide for yourself if expanding treatment, such as it is, makes sense.

How do the rehabs decide if you need treatment? I'll begin with the American Society of Addiction Medicine's (ASAM) criteria for admission to drug and alcohol treatment. Remember, doctors think like scientists. We like numbers. The doctors at ASAM did their best to try to organize just how bad a person is and how bad off things are with their addiction.

Their range is from zero (0) to four (IV). Zero is you're fine, have a nice day. A four (IV) and you need a hospital because your life is acutely in danger. Lower acuity scores (I-III) denote mild to more serious dependence. Thoughtfully, they'll assign a score of one-half (0.5), for those barely in the grip of substance habits.

If the addiction professionals think outpatient services will do, you are designated a I. Next is intensive outpatient (IOP) or partial hospitalization services (II to II.5). That goes up to residential inpatient services at level III. Three and a half (III.5) is clinically managed high-intensity residential services. Four (IV) is medically managed inpatient, intensive service. Those are sick people, typically in extremis from whatever the substance is, (i.e. cirrhosis) or withdrawal with risk of seizure. Sometimes a person has a bad problem with more than one substance. This is called creatively, polysubstance disorder. The drug causing the biggest problems for the patient weights the severity score the most.

For most people in treatment trying to come off a drug, they'll be designated at one of the higher levels, such as clinically managed high intensity residential services (III.5). As they detox and feel better, their level of acuity falls, back through residential, and then intensive outpatient, and then outpatient. The principle is a continuum, so the worse you are, the more help you need. The better off you are, the less support, care, and expense you need.

This also lines up with how insurance companies reimburse for addiction treatment services. The typical modern rehab will try to keep a customer in the highest level of care as long as possible because the reimbursement rates are the richest. Often, it's several thousand dollars a day for being in detox. Drug rehab is a $42 billion a year industry in the U. S., and going up.

While you may not yet be all better, by the time they kick you down a level, it usually means you have hit the limit of what your insurance policy will pay. Bear in mind that paying for addiction treatment can be as great a problem as the addiction itself. Fraud and abuse are rampant in the industry. "Body brokers" receive an undisclosed referral fee for sending an insured patient to a rehab. The kickbacks alone can run into five figures.

Utilization specialists at the rehab billing offices know the intimate details of insurance company payment criteria. As expert advisors, they coach the rehab clinicians on the proper language for maximum reimbursement. It's good business. The criteria for addiction severity are the language used by insurance company representatives to restrict reimbursement for care. Nearly all addiction treatment is organized on this reimbursement structure. Even the standard length of treatment programs is derived from insurance company guidelines.

When insurance benefits first began paying for drug and alcohol treatment in the 1980s, health insurance companies understandably freaked out. With up to one-fifth of their insured having a substance abuse problem at some point in their lives. They had to mitigate risk of huge payouts or risk financial collapse. Anne Fletcher in her excellent book, *Inside Rehab*, traces the origin of the thirty-day treatment paradigm.

Nobody really knows for sure, as the custom isn't based on any published document or scientific research. It appears to be a negotiated compromise between Hazelden, a rehab in Minnesota, that treated alcoholics in the 1950s, and the then newly formed health insurance companies. Back then, it took an alcoholic about a week or two in detox to feel okay. Two or three more weeks was the limit of coverage for an expensive inpatient stay. Obviously, addiction severity and robustness of individual coping and support vary widely; one-size-fits-all doesn't make sense. My hunch is we built the guidelines for care (ASAM criteria) to follow insurance company rules.

With abysmal long-term success rates only one month after of inpatient rehab discharge (and a scandalous 95 percent relapse within one year), treatment centers brazenly argued, for a longer course of care. Additional services and treatment methods were bolted on to the existing model. We now have many fine gradations, including outpatient, extended care, and so forth. The most expensive "celebrity" rehabs will even send a "sober companion" home with a customer. This isn't covered by insurance, and costs can run to hundreds if not thousands of dollars per day.

Intensive outpatient therapy (IOP) is ~15 hours a week, broken up over three days. It typically includes of a process group led by a counselor and, for some IOPs, they'll throw in an individual therapy session. If you're not meeting with a counselor, then you'll do some other "recovery related" activity. This can be movie watching, art therapy, career counseling, or whatever the individual program deems valuable. "Evidence-based" is a buzzword in treatment–allegedly indicating more than opinion recommends a particular therapy–and it's rarely more than lip-service as it pertains to efficacy.

Activities in rehab are structured and, might be mistaken for time-fillers to justify the cost of the outpatient program. Afterwards, most recommend or offer ongoing or continuing care, with periodic visits either with a counselor, or tagging up with the members of the therapy team from rehab. Substance abuse treatment of this kind mimics a treatment course for a *physical ailment* or an injury. Big intervention followed by graded increase in activity and clinic visits after rehab; same as if you had your appendix out, or recovered from a broken leg. Little by little, stronger and stronger, until you're all better.

Does this match your own personal experience that of someone you care about who tried to get sober? It typically takes years for a person's life to break down so badly that they qualify for a high level of care. I've yet to hear about an addict who went rehab the day after a *first* drink. Even people on heroin take a long time to degrade their lives such that treatment is urgent.

Most who try opiates (heroin included) never become addicted. Only 10 to 20 percent will need some kind of external support or treatment. It takes at least months and, more likely, years of use before they need to be in a hospital or a residential treatment facility. The idea that after a month of living in a (sometimes beautiful, often crummy) care home will result in someone reliably sorting out his problems is absurd. It sounds crazy, doesn't it? It does to me. Why is the rehab system, as implemented, still with us?

It takes far longer than a month even to get a handle on the real problem. Drugs and alcohol, though damaging and a significant issue in their own right, are really symptoms of a deeper issue. Substance habits seem take on a life of their own, but they are not primary. Nobody is born alcohol deficient. A major drawback that comes from going away to sequestered treatment is you don't get to work on the mundane causes of your emotional pain. These are what drive us to seek relief in drugs and drink. While you are away in rehab, your "inbox" fills up with all the questions, unopened mail, relationship problems, festering resentments, and regular business from your usual life.

Meanwhile, you're at the treatment facility sitting in group, going to "family" meals and, in nearly all rehabs, shuttling to 12-step recovery meetings. Primarily what you learn in a residential treatment setting is how to manage the bizarre ritual of being in treatment. You don't really learn how to deal with what comes up next in the real world, because those problems haven't yet reached your emotional shore. They're still far off in the future.

To overcome the habit of drinking and using, you have to create a new set of dynamically adapting responses. They are created by developing a new need-action-reward cycle. In other words, you need a replacement habit for dealing with your feelings.

In the last of your four weeks in a typical rehab (before your insurance runs out), if you're not too fuzzy from the near-ubiquitous psychiatric meds, you feel a sense of growing dread about returning to your old life. You know you were poorly equipped to manage the tangle of problems before rehab. The group therapy and community meals didn't give you many new tools. It's hard to deal with life as it comes, especially without the old crutch of drugs or alcohol.

If you are in a Seroquel®, or other "sleep med" fog, you probably won't resist the rehab counselor's advice to you stay a few weeks longer. Of course, only if you or your insurance company can afford it. Likely, your family and loved ones are encouraging you to stay.

Instead of the anxious and uncertainty knotting up in their stomachs, your family feels a sense of relief that you are "making good decisions" or "fighting your disease." You are scared of the outside world and hide in the rehab, loved ones (stakeholders in your success) don't have to deal with your antics while you are in a structured setting. Maybe your counselors are tiptoeing along the edge of client manipulation for "your own good." All of this is under the banner of saving you from a deadly disease. Since a third party is paying (insurance), there really is no rush to leave, right?

The rehab industry, it should come as no surprise, will tell you that staying in a treatment setting longer is better. Officially, they mean any treatment setting. Since residential care is intended to treat a higher level of addiction severity, the treatment people will try to convince you that not only is longer better, but the longer you can remain at a high acuity level, the better still. This advice is almost always conditioned on your financial resources or, if you have them, unused insurance benefits.

There is good evidence to assert that the longer a person is engaged in some kind of effort to deal with his substance habit issue, the better. This is just another way of saying people need time grow out of their self-destructive habits. It has never been shown in a good scientific study that the longer a person resides *in a treatment facility*, the more likely he is to remain sober after departure.

The notion that longer engagement with self-improvement leads to better chances at behavior modification is true, and duh, obvious. But if longer means sequestered, or hidden away from life, this isn't per se better. Rehab itself is no panacea. In my experience, it can even make you feel worse about yourself if you don't improve your ability to deal with reality. It is essential to be honest with yourself. By definition, living behind the walls of an institution is not the same as your real life.

People do, as a matter of the natural history of substance habits, spontaneously quit drinking/using. This happens at a baseline rate of around three percent (3%) per year. They just stop. Who knows why? If they were in rehab when they happened to quit for good, rehab gets the credit. We all use the availability heuristic (we explain the world with the concepts we have) and assign praise to the rehab for our success. Though the undesired outcome doesn't apply: it's on you if you relapse. The rehabs take credit for your success, but disavow responsibility for your failures. If you "fail" rehab (relapse to resume using), the facility will surely blame you and say, "he wasn't ready."

Some people do benefit from a brief period of separation from their drug-using routines. Certain environments are very difficult from which to escape the subconscious cues and prompts to drink or use. As mentioned, physical illness from the substances, their consequences (trauma, HIV, etc.), or dangerous withdrawal, all call for competent medical care. This subset of the truly ill is a minority of those addicted to drugs or alcohol. Despite the scary commercials for rehab, most people do not need this level of care to stop using. The average person with a substance habit can stop, he just has trouble staying stopped.

Most treatment facilities or rehabs are voluntary. Few are compelled by the bench. Although if a judge offers a man in his court the option of treatment (diversion) or jail, the accused usually picks rehab. There are inpatient jail treatment programs, but even there, inmate participation is voluntary. Prisoners who enroll in these treatment programs motivated by a mixture of genuine desire for sobriety and favorable treatment by the parole board. Self-interest reigns supreme. Another blow against the addiction-is-disease concept.

The bottom line is this: whether someone volunteers to go into rehab or a jail treatment program, or whether they are forced to get help because of an ultimatum, legal pressure, or some other reason, the results are usually the same – which, as you'll read in the next chapter, aren't good.

☐

–10–
TYPICAL TREATMENT OUTCOME

Treatment for addiction in America is generally ineffective. This fact is the elephant in the room for the whole industry. When challenged with the dismal success data, the standard response from traditional rehab proponents is either something about reducing stigma with calls for *more* treatment.

The data on successful treatment outcomes are very hard to come by. Most places either don't keep track of their success ratios, or they outright lie about their outcomes. If they do keep track, they don't want to share the raw data publicly. Mostly because the price of rehab is sky high and results are embarrassingly dismal. The failure data are guarded more tightly than Asa Candler's drink recipe in the safe at Coca-Cola headquarters.

When I say the results are poor, I'm talking single digit success numbers. Less than one in ten are abstinent at one year post rehab– and that is *by self-report*. If any legitimate follow-up at all is conducted, it typically entails calling people on the phone and asking them how they're doing. The responses vary as you might expect. Hardly anyone answering these phone surveys has been continuously abstinent since discharge. Some have moved, others are deceased. They usually tally no news as good news, leaving the MIA customers out of totals completely. Not s failure if they can't find you, right?

Response rates are low and people are embarrassed to admit "failure." Granted, some go to rehab with the intent of controlling their drinking/using afterward. I know of no rehab which tells people this is their intended goal (honestly, for those who get to the "need rehab" stage, abstinence is usually the best call, but that's up to you to decide). Rehabs usually claim you'll remain sober after discharge, but this result is uncommon.

Despite that, believe it or not, there is a treatment facility in Malibu, California that advertises a jaw-dropping 84 percent success rate. They don't define success except to say, "You'll be cured." Interestingly, despite having been open for two decades, their success rate has never changed year to year. It's always been 84 percent, from the first victim customer to the time of this writing. Why mess with success, right? Unscrupulous people will tell you anything just to make a buck when you're in a vulnerable position. After you have witnessed the ravages of a substance habit in a loved one, or experienced for yourself the misery of addiction, they tell you what you want to hear.

The tens of thousands of dollars you will spend, or for which your insurance company is about to be billed, is all done in the name of saving a life. They claim it is going to work "if you work it." By implication, they provide the healing, and any failure inures to you. Nothing really could be further from the truth as treatment usually fails.

This is not to take away from the success stories, but they are a fraction of each group of "graduates." Most people relapse soon after discharge from treatment. Rudolph and Bernice Moos, in a study from 2006 published in the research journal *Addiction*, noted that up to 90 percent of *treated* alcoholics relapse.

The best data on success rates I've seen for a traditional treatment facility come from a Hazelden/Betty Ford report. The most recent data I've seen is from 2008, but I have no reason to think they're any different today. "The Betty" admits only a fifty-fifty chance of abstinence at one year.[1] Bear in mind, though, if the aftercare department couldn't reach somebody by

---

[1] Consumer's Digest, 2008

phone, they noted the patient as "lost to follow-up." Many rehabs will record that result as "sober." On average, their graduates are still drinking/using, embarrassed to have gone to rehab, and many thousands of dollars poorer. It is no wonder the treatment facilities won't share their data: their business model would be pulverized if the truth got out.

A major component of treatment in rehab facilities is, medication. Unfortunately, medication for addiction habits has a terrible track record; people swap the new drug in place of the old. Remember the plight of Dr. Halstead? He switched from cocaine to heroin. The results weren't good. Barbiturate sedatives, prescribed as far back as the 1920s, have a bad history too. In the 1960s, a breakthrough class of "safe" medications called benzodiazepines received FDA approval. The flagship drug, Valium, was prescribed as a promise for alcoholics and their "anxiety."

It was a disaster for patients with substance habits. This has also been the case with every so-called "non-addictive" medication that has abuse potential. A classic is Ambien, one of the "Z" drugs. Ambien pill that isn't a benzodiazepine until you take it (liver turns the pro-drug into a benzo). As a consequence of repeated pharmaceutical failures, most people in the recovery world are hesitant to embrace substitute medications – especially the sort that blur consciousness. Researchers still seek the holy grail of addiction treatment: a drug that cures the problem without creating another problem.

Most of the medical studies used by the FDA to approve new drugs rely on a standard you may not have seen. They look for a reduction in the "total number of heavy drinking days." If a new medicine, on average, can reduce the heavy drinking days in a month from, say, *twenty-four* to *twenty-one*, then that drug is categorized as useful and good, even though for the accepted canons on the industry, lack of abstinence would denote failure. That would be three fewer *heavy* drinking days a month, while still having three solid weeks as a lush. You have to be careful about the drug industry's criteria for success, but improvement is improvement. I predict you'll see less emphasis in the years ahead on abstinence and more on reduction in substance habits.

Another issue is trying to treat a habit problem with medication alone. The principal thesis of this book is addiction is an elaborate habit. As such, it cannot be eradicated with a medication or single intervention. Habit formation and maintenance take time and are complex phenomena. When we try and fix a complex problem like an alcohol habit with a single medication, we're bound to experience poor results. Proper medication with a structured program for habit change is probably the state-of-the-art in support for substance addiction.

A good example of a failed "magic bullet" when used in isolation is Acamprosate or Campral®, which is prescribed to heavy drinkers so they'll stop drinking. A Cochrane report (a method of combining several low-power studies to answer the question, *Does this work?*) from 2010 by Rösner[2], et. al, answered that question. Their conclusion, after combining twenty-four Campral® studies, is plain:

"Even though the sizes of treatment effects appear to be rather moderate in their magnitude, they should be valued against the background of the relapsing nature of alcoholism and the limited therapeutic options currently available for its treatment."

In other words, "We don't have much to offer and at least this doesn't seem to hurt." The key measurement is NNT, or Number Needed to Treat. In the case of Campral®, the NNT is over *nine*. That means eight of nine people get no benefit but have to take the medication three times a day anyway. One in nine Acamprosate-takers reports benefit, but *objective* measures (lab tests) like liver function (GGT) suggest people are pounding the cocktails same as ever on the Acamprosate. Medication alone, and I'm looking at you too M.A.T., won't ever work.

In my own practice, however, I prescribe Acamprosate differently than just writing a script. In my experience, Campral® is best used a *part of* a comprehensive habit change program. As monotherapy, it is very unimpressive. When combined with an education, support and

---

[2] Cochrane Database Syst Rev. 2010 Sep 8;(9):CD004332. doi: 10.1002/14651858.CD004332.pub2.
Acamprosate for alcohol dependence.

Rösner S1, Hackl-Herrwerth A, Leucht S, Lehert P, Vecchi S, Soyka M.
Author information
1
Psychiatric Hospital, University of Munich, Nussbaumstr. 7, Munich, Germany, 80336.

accountability regimen, it is remarkably helpful at reducing the urge to drink.

The current monthly average pharmacy cost for Campral® is around $300: a small price to pay for better traction in your habit change program. And far less than the least expensive rehab I know of. Be aware though, simply taking Campral® without real change in your routine and habit patterns likely won't lead to abstinence. But if you're establishing a new habit practice aimed at curbing alcohol or benzodiazepine usage, you might find Campral® very helpful. Since it requires a prescription, see your doctor.

Let's look again at treatment facilities *if* they report their success rates at all, they report success in the vaguest terms. If you went to treatment graduated, relapsed, stayed wasted for months, and then spent the night in a holding cell for drunk & disorderly, incidentally sobering up the day before, and you happened to get a phone call from your rehab and they asked, "are you drinking?" Of course, you responded, "I'm sober." That counts as a success – for the *rehab*.

Also, if you relapsed multiple times, had a really bad go of it for a number of years, maybe went to several other different treatment facilities, and then finally managed to stop, then the first treatment facility will consider you their success (we got him started on the right path), as will every facility you attended along the way. In other words, we really can't trust anything that comes out of the treatment facilities because they don't have standard criteria for success. It's not in their financial or marketing interest. In fact, one of the dirty secrets of the rehab industry is "keep coming back."

Naturally, there can be merit in going back for more help. But just because treatment failed doesn't mean you should go back again and again. This premise has gone largely unchallenged in the treatment industry. There are two reasons for this. Health of the rehab industry is one. The other is the uncomfortable truth that we don't really know how to help someone, and the risk of failing to "fix" the addict is possible death.

If we administer treatment for any other problem, such as diabetes or pneumonia, the same way rehabs run, we'd be out of business before we started. If your pneumonia treatment cost $30,000 and had a 10 percent chance of success, you'd probably ask for a different treatment, a different doctor. Or call a priest to administer last rites. But because people don't have the information before they come in for treatment, they are at a lopsided disadvantage. They don't know what they bought until after treatment ends.

At least when you buy a car it has wheels, an engine, and you can test drive it. If the car is missing one or more of those features it will be plain to see before you take delivery. When you buy treatment, you don't really know what you're getting. You don't know how long it's going to last. You don't know if it's going to work. And I hate to sound even more depressing than I do, but most of addiction treatment is set up *to fail.* You'll hear in rehab that *relapse is part of recovery.* That's like saying pneumonia progressing to empyema is part of the treatment for pneumonia. Pure bunkum.

So, what does work? In terms of raw numbers, people get help for their substance use most commonly through their place of worship. They go to organized religious services and meet with their spiritual advisors for help. Help with their family, financial, or social issues. This is what rabbis, priests, pastors, ministers, imams, and monks are in the business of doing. Addiction is often characterized as a spiritual malady marked by "straying" from the path. Some of the better faith-based organizations have created ongoing programs that integrate the tenets and rituals of their particular religion to support people in early recovery.

Former Health, Education and Welfare Secretary, Joseph Califano,[3] decried the lack of coordination between clergy and doctors. Today, seventy million Americans or more are grappling with substance abuse, and another one hundred million know someone who needs help. Ninety-five percent of those polled believe in God or some sort of spirituality, but psychiatrists don't generally recommend their patients speak with their own clergy. It's a missed opportunity. As AA notes, we should be quick to see where religious people are right.

What other solutions have we for the vexing problem of a substance habit? There is one approach that has over decades proven to be the most successful for helping people transition from substance habits to a

---

3

FEBRUARY 11, 2002 ISSUE
Religion, Science and Substance Abuse
 Joseph A. Califano, Jr.
February 11, 2002

substance-free life. It is the program I went through called diversion. To land in the most successful treatment program ever devised was just luck on my part. Simply because I am a physician, the diversion program was offered to me when I needed to quit fentanyl. It works approximately nine out of ten times; rehab works for only one person out of ten. How can this be? First, let me share with you a little history on treating doctors who are addicted instead of arresting them.

As we discussed earlier in this book, in the 1970s, thousands of veterans fighting in Vietnam had become addicted to heroin. Compassionate voices called for treatment and rehabilitation of the young soldiers. Hard-bitten realists agreed: there were too many to ignore. In the same spirit of helping the helpers, caring for our fighting forces sparked an interest in the mental health of our domestic physician corps.

There a landmark article in the *Journal of the American Medical Association* in 1974, which detailed the history of physicians who developed an addiction to drugs or alcohol.

The radical idea was to *treat* physicians who get sick, instead of yanking their licenses. This was a watershed moment and it led to treatment for all kinds of "squishy" issues, including depression, anxiety, declining physical skills, burn-out, and suicide. It's clear a surgeon ought to be able to see, hear, and use her hands in order to do a good job. Reluctant at first to admit they were human too, doctors eventually were the vanguard of a revolution in mental health.

As an outgrowth, California started the Medical Board Diversion Program. The crux: instead of bouncing doctors out of medical practice because they developed a substance habit, let's instead offer them treatment and a path to rehabilitation. Instead of kicking them out of medicine and taking their license, essentially saying "beat it," California started putting them in treatment. Besides the humane angle, it was good fiscal policy for the State. An individual doctor treated thousands of citizens per year and improved bottom-line GDP in California so much, the state could ill afford losing many physicians to a treatable problem.

Also, a pioneer program in Los Angeles was started by gastroenterologist-turned-addiction-doctor David Murphy. "Murph" was sober and public about it. These new mental health/diversion groups started treating doctors with the best help they could find. At the time, modalities included group and individual talk therapy, peer support, worksite monitoring, and drug testing. With the first few docs choosing recovery over resignation, by 1980, the California Physician Health Program, or Diversion Program was underway. The first two-year data were astonishing: eight out of ten doctors were sober and back to work. Only two kept drinking and turned in their licenses.

As word of their success spread, more doctors were referred into Diversion. As hospital boards and administrators witnessed the first hundred success stories, including drugs as well as alcohol, many hospital administrative directors joined the diversion movement to support the next wave of doctors coming through. The premise was sound, and the tracking and follow up were nearly perfect. For example, drug testing sample collection, was *directly observed*. A same-sex monitor watched participants urinate in a sample cup so there was no opportunity for sample mix-up or shenanigans.

Diversion was eventually replicated in all fifty states. Two significant research papers, one from the original, California Diversion Program, and later one from the Washington State Physicians Health Program, confirmed long-term excellent results. 85% to 95% is the observed likelihood of documented abstinence at the end of a five-year program. Truly astonishing success for an otherwise intractable problem.

The State Diversion Programs became the model for the country's doctors, and the strategy was adopted internationally. Later, the same principles would be applied to programs for nurses and pharmacists. They worked for pilots and attorneys, too. The common theme was helping individuals with substance habit who work in a position of public trust.

As these programs spread, they yielded data on participant outcome. The findings are not merely based on a telephone call asking the doctor if he is sober. The aim is not a reduction in the total number of heavy drinking days. These are verified urine drug-screen negative, and meeting all the other the criteria in terms of proper professional behavior. Unambiguous, objective evidence of abstinence was required, or participants wouldn't be allowed to work. Public safety was the primary concern, but the programs figured out how to align the physician's health with the public trust: the doc had to be sober.

Initially, they required two-year minimum participation, this was gradually lengthened. The California Medical board observed a low relapse rate, but it dropped even lower after two years. Another "shoulder" in the success curve was at three years. So, for good measure, programs in most states lengthened to five years. Better safe than sorry.

The "carrot" in Diversion is not only a resumption of livelihood that comes with a safe return to medical practice, but a true second chance. If a physician signs up voluntarily and completes all requirements, their entire Diversion file is tossed in the shredder. For docs who are not voluntary participants, and in some programs, the board hangs onto the file, just in case. If they do the right thing for five years, they get the benefit of grace. It's as if they never had a problem in the eyes of the state board.

Of course, they still have to be sober, they still have to behave, and it's strongly suggested to them that they not return to drinking or using drugs in any form or amount because it tends to lead to recrudescence of the original problem. Remember, Diversion can't shield a doc from legal problems or civil lawsuits. The second chance is only for keeping a license, not avoiding discipline or malpractice claims.

Most doctors who complete the entire five years remain sober from there on. Four point five out of five, in the California Diversion outcome data, and five out of six in the Washington study. Contrast this with thirty-day rehab programs and their success rate of, max, 10%. Compare that to the Diversion Program's eight in ten or better rate; there's no contest. If we could do it, we should have *everyone*, doctors and kings and janitors, do a diversion-style program.

For those who don't succeed in the diversion program, the State Medical Board will deem the doctor a public safety risk and take away the license. This is right and proper, as the proper role of the State is public safety, and practicing medicine is a privilege.

Given the typical treatment outcome for non-doctors (non-pilots, etc.) is so bad, and the physician treatment outcome is excellent, what accounts for the difference? It's not because doctors are any different or special, or they somehow have a milder form of the problem. They don't. Take it from me, the way doctors drink and use is the same as everybody else with these habits. It's the accountability, the community support (same boat), and above all the *duration*, which combine to make the difference. It takes a long time to change an old habit.

There is an alternative explanation for the dramatic difference in success between Diversion and regular rehab. Becoming a doctor requires a huge investment in time and money. Once training is complete, the rewards are great to the doctor in terms of job satisfaction, social status, and remuneration. It is a hard job to walk away from, especially if you have a family to support.

For doctors who come to the attention of physician health programs they are given a choice like I was: join this monitoring program and complete it successfully, or surrender your license and stop being a doctor. Severe? Yes, of course. But it may be part of the outstanding success rate. Doctors are told they can remain in good standing if they toe the line. Nearly all of us take the deal.

If doctors can change their "diseased" behavior with a contingency management system as described here (stay sober or get a different career), then maybe the way to treat substance habits is with the motivation of a big goal. If you want to help somebody achieve something great, you need to help them see the promise and help them pay the price. The promise of a new life, free from the negative downward pull of substance habits, and the price of not using even when you feel like it, are the twin pillars of any successful program.

China-sourced fentanyl, drug cartels based in Mexico, and diverted prescriptions are all major components of the opioid crisis. But the biggest cause of the opioid disaster in the U.S. is a lack of hope. Diversion-style programs would help anyone if we could capture the attention of those embroiled with the prospect of a better future. Remember, pain perception is relative. Less pain = more pleasure. The challenge in convincing those with substance habits to discipline themselves. The payoff is a new set of habits which will dynamically see them through the next round of challenges – and the one after that.

These programs have been applied to other high-leverage situations where public safety's important–airline pilots, attorneys, nurses, pharmacists, and law enforcement–and they've had similar success rates to the doctor cohort. Most of the benefits from Diversion programs accrue in the first three years. If we're going to take this problem seriously, we have to think beyond the 30-day + aftercare model. In a culture of expedient pleasure & relief, how to keep addicts plugged into the program for the long haul?

Putting them in a residential setting with sound baths and private chefs, like many of the Malibu rehabs, seems ideal. Add legal drugs and they will probably stay a second month if they can afford to. But this is unsustainable for five years. Longer term treatment in residential treatment is not better in terms of success results. Diminishing returns set in after only a week or two. It also can't work because a main challenge of participating in these programs is the relentless march of life, *while you're busy trying to make new habits*. You have events unfolding back home, issues at work, anxiety, stress, and the day-to-day strain of life. The in-box fills up whilst you're away.

The quotidian issues everyone has to deal with in order to get by don't take a break while you're in rehab. Not grabbing a drink, pill, toke, or shot when life takes a twist, how you handle life when it's challenging, those are the real hallmarks of conquering your habit.

Sober in rehab is a pitiful standard for treatment success. Most rehabs struggle to meet even this low bar. But to make it on the 'natch outside, and you'll have to figure out other ways of dealing with fear, frustration, and eventually with success. Thus, if we could bring this long-term, low-level Diversion-style treatment to everyone, we could make an enormous impact on addiction worldwide.

To solve the opioid epidemic in America, we should consider a 1930s-style massive public works program. We can put our idle men and women, shut out by globalization's off-shoring of their jobs, back to work—perhaps on the nation's crumbling infrastructure. Or they could learn to code, or become entrepreneurs. Some they could take one of the millions of open skilled jobs which don't require a college degree. This will not only help the country be ready for the future of transportation, information technology, and energy transmission, but it will give a generation of addicts a meaningful endeavor. They can participate in the building of a legacy and acquire valuable training and experience. That's the carrot.

The stick? They have to remain sober and subject to drug testing during their participation in the project. What if judges suspended sentences and offered the convicted a shot at a better life? Let's do for everyone what we do for physicians. Everyone has value and can be redeemed through effort and by mutual support and love. And no there's no shame in struggling. It's hard to make changes these big in your life. Get back up, brush yourself off and start again. You haven't failed until you quit trying.

Myself and a team of really smart tech professionals are working on an app, called VHAB (vhab.com), which is built on the principles of the Diversion systems discussed here. Community, education, and accountability, and time are the core principles of any successful habit change program. We've built the platform to help substance habit folks at the fun-with-problems stage.

At this stage, drinking/using isn't all, or always, fun. Sometimes it goes great, other days it's a shit show. Trouble is, it becomes harder to predict drink to drink, whether you're getting the fun or the problems. You're not bad enough to go to rehab, but you need to do something affordable and private about your habit. Check out VHAB. Download it from the app store if you're curious.

In the next few chapters, we'll get into the specifics of particular drugs and the way a typical detox course goes. Standard disclaimers apply here because everyone is a unique individual. Nothing contained in this book, or anywhere on any website I'm connected with in any way, constitutes specific medical advice for your situation. I'm a doctor but I'm not *your* doctor.

These are broad overarching ideas about how typical cases go. Your case may not be typical. See a doctor in person. So, with these caveats in mind let's talk about specific drugs. The list includes alcohol, opiates, marijuana, sedatives (or benzodiazepines, like Valium), and amphetamines.

–11–
ALCOHOL AND DETOX

Eighty million years ago our primate ancestors ate rotting fruit and got sick from the ethanol it contained. Ten million years ago, one lucky monkey was born with a mutation allowing it to break down alcohol. We carry that mutation, the ADH4 gene today. Alcohol has been used in ceremonies since the dawn of civilization. Stale beer residue in the bottom of old clay jars from along the Yellow River dates back 9,000 years ago, confirming brewing for deliberate intoxication. Some say the earliest civilization found in Anatolia, Turkey at the Gobekli Tipi, was formed to ferment grain for alcohol, not make bread for food. In any case, people have an ancient social and biological relationship to alcohol.

Humans detoxify and clear alcohol primarily in the liver. Technically, its metabolism actually begins in the mouth as alcohol is absorbed across the lining of the oral mucosa. Ethanol, the chemical name for potable alcohol, is also one of the few drugs absorbed directly through the wall of the stomach. Most others are not absorbed until farther down the gut at the small intestine. The reason I mention this is the rapid absorption of alcohol contributes to its potential to be habit-forming. The *rate of rise* of the blood level of a drug is what causes the feeling of a rush.

Alcohol is a very small molecule made of two carbons, six hydrogens, and one oxygen atom. No one knows exactly how it makes us drunk, or what it does in the brain. There are some studies that tell us how it works on the nerves: by slowing them down. Alcohol is a sedative; it depresses neural function. Depressed neural function just means that the nerves don't work like normal.

At this point, most people wonder, "If alcohol is a sedative, then how come when I drink it I feel more like talking or dancing or interacting with other people?" All of a sudden, it's not as intimidating to talk to potential romantic partners. Inhibitions are lifted, and that's the key right there. It's the inhibitory circuits of the brain, the cautionary parts that usually say "Don't do that. Be careful. Don't let anyone see you. Don't make a fool of yourself," that are inhibited first. This is why alcohol has been described as a social lubricant. It loosens us up by inhibiting self-control.

The first part of the brain to be sedated is the frontal lobe. This "judgment center" is usually the chaperone for most behavior. Party time. Usually drinking makes us more gregarious and bolder. Liquid courage. As a side note, this is probably why human beings drink alcohol, and it's probably why they use drugs in general. With decreased inhibition, we take more risks.

From an evolutionary standpoint, it's an advantage to the *population* of human beings if at least a few members take on extra risk. True, an individual risk-taker may have a shortened lifespan. The mysterious noise outside the cave may be coming from something that makes you its meal. On the other hand, that sound may be a new source of food. So, risk taking is potentially beneficial to the group, so long as everyone doesn't run outside and get eaten. Obviously, putting one's entire species on a single turn of the wheel is not a good strategy, and addiction doesn't seem to work that way. Some people have more propensity than others to take risk.

Anyhow, back to alcohol. The part of the brain that is inhibited first is the inhibitory, but then eventually the rest of the brain joins the Mardi Gras. Alcohol delays nerve transmission, thereby making it harder for the nerves to carry information. You may have had that experience if you've ever been buzzed or drunk. Everything's a little bit harder to do. Motor impairment is a hallmark of alcohol's effects. We don't (usually) drink to become uncoordinated. That's an unavoidable side effect. We drink to turn down the inhibitory tone of our risk-averse minds.

As I mentioned before, the brain is adaptive and very good at adapting to tolerate a sedative (alcohol). The brain adjusts its sensitivity the same way that you might turn up your speakers: to better hear a quiet part of a song.

Or turn them down for a loud commercial on television. The brain dials up the sensitivity to compensate for the suppressive effects of the chemical alcohol. By the way, this applies to all the sedatives. The nerves don't work as readily in the presence of a sedative, so gain ramps up. Receptors get more sensitive, or there are more of them present at the places where cells talk with each other (synapses).

If alcohol is taken away when the brain and nervous system are used to having it around, the receptors fire at a much higher rate and with much less stimulus required to make them fire. Information that is not supposed to be transmitted is transmitted. The neurons make up a story about what's going on.

This over-amplification underpins the phenomenon of hallucinations when someone is detoxing from alcohol. DTs, or *delirium tremens* are hallucinations and anxiety often accompanied by trembling or shaking. Delirium, from the Latin for "plowing outside of the furrow." Tremens is from the French for "shaking" or "trembling." The neurons of the brain and nervous system are so twitchy in alcohol withdrawal, that they can fire in groups. We observe the effects of these spontaneous firings as shaking, jerky movements.

Remember, the brain's job is to organize the world, to infer patterns, to sort the vital from the irrelevant. When the sensitivity levels are adjusted really high, the pattern formation (our recognition of what's what), is altered. In this case, we start seeing and sensing patterns where there aren't any. This can lead to things like paranoia, anxiety, or plain old fear. Bad cases of withdrawal can even lead to seizure. If you've been drinking for a while, your mind knows full well that the next drink will take away a lot of that anxiety and discomfort. You could say it's a habit and you wouldn't be wrong.

That's really what craving is. Craving is just a thought that seems really important because we focus on it and overvalue it. That's the nature of all perception. The things that we're focused on seem to be the ones that are the most important at that time. The mind's primary function is to sort out the useful from the useless. It is axiomatic that the object or idea upon which we focus must be important: *why else focus on it?*

Once you've been exposed to alcohol for a while, the brain adapts to its presence. When you stop, the brain in effect says "hey, where's my alcohol?" and that is manifested as a feeling of craving. Even more pernicious is the craving for control of your *internal* environment. We don't actually want the booze (drug, whatever) but rather, we crave the feeling of control and the reduction of uncertainty that repetitive habitual using affords.

Granted, craving thoughts seem especially intense and clamor for your immediate attention. Make no mistake though. Craving does not distinguish the "alcoholic" from "normal people." Everyone has experienced intense desire for something (or someone) that is fed by the habitual reward expected and, more fundamentally, by the attention we pay to the thought itself. For most people with a compulsive idea to use drugs or drink when they are detoxing, redirecting the attention away from the craving for as little as one minute will usually "break the spell." Don't linger over the idea of drinking or using while you are trying to quit. Reminiscing about the good old days is one of the worst things you can do. Get out of the barbershop—unless you want a haircut.

The elevated nerve transmission discussed above, lead to an increased sensitivity for seizure. Because the brain, habituated to alcohol, has to go without, its function is revved-up compared to baseline. The brain is extra sensitive, and the little electric signals that pass between neurons can sometimes get amplified to the point where they fire uncontrollably. This is a seizure.

When a seizure is triggered, brain damage can occur from the spike in metabolic consumption by the neurons. And because a seizure causes one to lose control of the body, there is also the risk of trauma if you are driving, or atop a ladder when the seizure occurs. A seizure can also make you bite your tongue or vomit.

Of all the drugs, except for benzodiazepines (which we'll cover later), alcohol withdrawal is the most dangerous. Of deaths reported due to detox, alcohol is the most frequent, though still uncommon overall. Most people don't get to the point that their autonomic nervous systems are deeply suppressed by alcohol, thank God. It is not a good idea to abruptly stop drinking if you case is advanced. If you're drinking around the clock, especially in the morning, you should definitely see a doctor before just quitting.

Interestingly, opiates are among the lowest for detox-deaths, although people say the suffering from opiate withdrawal is the worst. Public perception is it's harder and more dangerous to kick opiates than alcohol, but medically that's not true. Opioid withdrawal is risky for people who go back to using because they lose tolerance and can easily overdose.

Part of the challenge with alcohol and its detox is the short duration of action of the substance itself. The shorter the duration of action of a drug, the more often the person needs to consume it or ingest it. The short-acting drugs have increased likelihood of eventual dependence. Also, because the alcohol only lasts for a few hours, the dosing interval is brief, minutes to hours.

Another way you can see this is in the pattern of the heavy drinker. See if this sounds familiar. He drinks throughout the day, earlier and earlier, year by year, as the habit progresses. This makes quitting hard because the nerve suppression of the last drink of alcohol only lasts a few hours. Drink #2 through #4 is the golden stretch. Not too drunk, but not in rough withdrawal either. The feelings of craving, anxiety, discomfort, paranoia, and fear that come along with alcohol withdrawal are staved off temporarily by the next drink.

As mentioned, for all drugs, the sensation of being high correlates with the rate of change in blood level. The rising blood level is the result of the substance increasing in amount in the bloodstream. It's as simple as that. The falling blood level is just the opposite. As the body metabolizes the substance, the blood level falls.

Our perception or sense of the effects a drug is most intense when it's rising in our blood. The increase moment to moment provides a sense of feeling high. The plateau of feeling comfortable that we seek, the stable perception of *just right,* is something you can never really get. It is always fleeting because the feeling of being high requires an increasing drug level.

The toxic and sedating effects in the case of alcohol or tranquilizers is reached *before* the steady state of having an unchanging blood level. Further, if you have a stable blood level, your brain and nervous system will adapt, and then you won't feel the *velocity* of getting high at all. Since the only way to remain high is to have a rising blood level, which is not permanently possible, you can never achieve that perfect state of nirvana. There is no way to stick a pin in the good times and have them last forever. Although I've repeatedly and unsuccessfully attempted it. Permanent relief from suffering by using substances is a state which can never be achieved.

How should we manage alcohol withdrawal? I again strongly recommend that you consult a live doctor, because the risk of alcohol withdrawal and even death are real, especially if you have other medical conditions and drink a lot. Death from alcohol toxicity or acute liver failure are not uncommon in the United States.

In my opinion, tragic is the person who decides to stop drinking and then is harmed by quitting itself. Almost everyone who is dependent on alcohol can be taken off safely.

To detox as safely as possible, doctors recommend drugs that allow moderate sedation, but without the toxicity of alcohol. The overall aim is to craft a regimen which allows for the transition from dependence to abstinence. Another approach, more popular with doctors in Europe, uses anti-seizure medications for alcohol detox. Elevation in heart rate and blood pressure, and seizures, are the big risks of alcohol withdrawal. Prevention of these effects, which an anti-seizure drug can help with, makes withdrawal much safer.

The best thing about these detox meds is they're not alcohol. Alcohol itself damages your tissues, including intestines, liver, brain, heart, and kidneys. Coupled with the effects of withdrawal, sometimes stopping is not so simple. The traditional way of managing alcohol withdrawal is to prescribe a sedative, usually a benzodiazepine, that flattens the acuity curve of your withdrawal symptoms. It just means that the severity or intensity of the withdrawal discomfort is lessened. Let me explain.

If you think about a curve that goes up, over, and back down; imagine a simple parabolic curve like the shape of the St. Louis arch. We'll say the total amount of discomfort that a person is going to experience when they withdraw (opiates, alcohol or sedatives) is represented by the cumulative area under the curve. For our arch example, it's all the open space under the big steel curve. How quickly we get to the peak, the *steepness* of increasing withdrawal symptoms, is the pain that oftentimes drives people back to drinking. The purpose of prescribing a benzodiazepine like Ativan for a person coming off alcohol, is to lower the peak of suffering. You all know now about flattening the curve from the COVID pandemic.

People ask, "doc, if I'm on this other drug, then doesn't that just prolong everything?" Yes, and it doesn't eliminate the total amount of discomfort or suffering that a person has to go through, but it does lower the peak. Most people will happily trade an extra day or two of moderate withdrawal discomfort, so long as worst of it is less bad. That is how most alcohol detox is accomplished. But another word about substances like

Valium or Ativan when is used for detox. They put a person at risk for developing dependence.

Unfortunately, many go to their doctor and complain of anxiety or stress, but they don't tell the medico about their alcohol use. If a patient complains about trouble sleeping; the doctor might prescribe a few days of a sleeping pill. If the insomniac takes sleeping pills and downs them with alcohol, she'll get hammered. Synergy, or $1 + 1 = 3$, forces the brain to adapt to the flood of sedation. If the troubled sleeper survives the cocktail of sedative and booze to develop a habit, she'll have extra difficulty when she stops.

If you're dependent on alcohol or sedatives, please be honest with your doctor, and don't drink *while* you're taking medication. You'll not only defeat the purpose, but also put yourself in danger. Benzodiazepines and sedatives have their place when prescribed correctly. They reduce the likelihood of seizure and make the discomfort of withdrawal more bearable. Combined with ethanol though, and you're playing with fire.

Flattening the suffering curve, is a compassionate, gentle, and safer way for dealing with alcohol withdrawal. Let's look at a few additional problems with alcohol detox, with an eye on long-term damage. Develop a dependence on alcohol and you ought to have blood work done. At minimum, you'll need a doctor to evaluate the status of your red blood cells and bone marrow. Alcohol is directly toxic to the factory for new blood cells housed inside the skeleton. Booze attacks two ways: by harming the mother cells which divide to create new blood, and also by inhibiting the absorption of key nutrients from the small intestine. The most common vitamin deficiency in drinkers is thiamine (vitamin B1).

Thiamine is essential for brain and overall neurologic health. Chronic low thiamine causes dementia. Its lack in heavy drinker was observed to be so common in Europe, distillers are required by law to add it to alcohol. It's less expensive for their national health care system to add the vitamin to hard spirits, than it is to treat wide-scale dementia or encephalopathy. As a public health harm-reduction strategy, rather than try to treat people once they become badly damaged by alcohol, they add vitamins to the whisky and other spirits.

In addition to blood work, you should get a physical exam, at least by telemedicine, because there is a risk of organ damage with alcohol consumption. Cirrhosis, a condition of liver tissue being replaced by scar tissue, can cause you to turn a certain shade of yellow. This is just one of the health issues possible from long-term drinking. A gastroenterology professor once described drinking alcohol as like internal chemical burns. He said if your liver had pain nerves like your fingertips do, you would never take a second drink; that's how toxic alcohol is to the body.

Alcohol is absorbed by the intestine. It is processed by and chemically damages the liver. If the damage is chronic and sustained, then the liver will become fibrous: a big pebbled scar. This is not good: healthy cells replaced with tough, lifeless collagen. Your liver is the filter and source of clotting factors for the whole body. If the liver stops working, it can lead to unchecked bleeding and malnutrition from poor protein synthesis (albumen).

With a scarred little liver blood can's pass through easily. Blood returning from the intestine backs up in the veins, and they swell with elevated pressure. Some of these veins (especially the ones near the esophagus) can bleed and lead to fatal hemorrhage. If you've ever thrown up blood, you know it's bad. Seek medical attention immediately if this is happening to you, because it may mean that you have cirrhosis (or early stages of it) and the veins are literally backing up along your esophagus. A little extra straining (vomiting) and those veins can tear. I've seen people bleed to death internally from this condition called portal hypertension. They didn't even know they were bleeding internally

A physical exam can also reveal yellow eyes, or icterus, which indicates the liver is having trouble processing the breakdown products of blood. We won't go into details about the physiology, but when old hemoglobin is eliminated, the liver does that job. When it can't, pigment starts to stick around in the body, and that can yellow the eyes. If any of these descriptions apply to you, then you should see a doctor as soon as possible (even if you haven't stopped drinking) because you may be putting yourself in significant danger of death. Assuming everything is okay physically, your doctor will recommend a treatment regimen for coming off alcohol, usually with a sedative.

Most people who go through this want to know if they can ever drink again. They remember fondly the good times and relaxed inhibitions that alcohol provided, forgetting the physical pain, terror, paranoia, and body damage that came later. This cycle of dependence, quitting, and relapse is very common. Chances are, you or someone you love has been through this cycle, probably many times.

The reason I wrote this book is I fell off the wagon myself many times before sobriety finally stuck. Repeatedly, I swore I'd never go back to drinking or using drugs, only to find myself caught up in it again. It was a slow-motion disaster. My day-to-day struggle to stop felt impossible. Any substance has a long-term cumulative effect to damage the brain and body, but that feels like tomorrow's problem. The short-term effect is escape from plaguing thoughts of self-doubt. I don't need to tell you how hard it is to stay away from it.

Here I cajole, urge and bullyrag you into getting a physician for your detox. Not only for safety reasons, but also, it's good practice simply to ask for help. This is something I struggled with, and continue to work on. For a long time, I was afraid to involve anyone else in my struggles because I didn't know what was going to happen. I thought I was going to be humiliated and embarrassed, and somehow if I admitted my habits, I would be irredeemable.

I learned later, everyone struggles with *something*; there's no such thing as a "normal person." Everyone has the tendency or proclivity to use or do some kind of repetitive behavior in order to manage his feelings. You are just like nearly everyone else if you prefer to avoid embarrassment in social settings. If you think you can manage something on your own, like most of us, you probably will try to. A company called Roman sells impotence and hair loss medication via mail with a video doctor visit. Another company called *Hims* does pretty much the same thing. They're enormously successful because their customers are embarrassed to discuss such personal struggles face-to-face. They provide a useful service to help people get started.

If you'd feel sheepish talking with a doctor, therapist or friend about your drinking or substance habit, that just makes you like everyone else. And it made me like everyone else, only I couldn't tell until *after* I got help.

In the next section, we will discuss opiate withdrawal, and since it is a national emergency, as proclaimed by President Trump, we'll give it special attention.

–12–
OPIATES AND DETOX

This is a subject which hits close to home as injectable opiates were the substance that forced me to choose between life and death. We've gone over my physical dependence on the super-potent opiate called fentanyl. Though strong, it is essentially the same as morphine-type drugs used throughout history. Socrates observed wheat and poppies grew together in the same field, surely a sign the gods intended pain relief as vital to man as food.

A word about terminology and definitions: opiates and opioids are used interchangeably in this text, though they're not precisely the same. Opiates are derivatives of the opium poppy (*Papaver somniferum*), which means sleep-bringing, and they include morphine, codeine, heroin, and others. These derivatives are extracts, or are byproducts of the opium plant. Drugs similar in chemical structure and effect, but that are *not* derived from the poppy, are called opioids. Opioids include things like hydrocodone, which you'd find in Vicodin, Norco, Dilaudid, and of course, fentanyl.

Probably the most notorious opioid in America, if not fentanyl, is oxycodone. Sold under the brand name OxyContin, it is pushed as a long-acting painkiller. Oxycodone in a regular pill, is a short-acting molecule–

maybe lasting four hours. Combined with a slow-release matrix in the structure of the OxyContin pill, it's more slowly absorbed and therefore lasts longer.

Oxycodone works at our opiate receptors and it reduces pain and suffering. Unfortunately, its short duration of action makes abuse and dependence more likely in premarketing studies. Intended to reduce addiction risk while at the same time increasing the pain reduction profile, Purdue created a longer duration medicine by delaying its absorption, nothing more. Yes, there are intrinsically long-acting opioids, and methadone is the prototype.

Methadone is an excellent *pain medicine* with a long duration of action, but it is most commonly prescribed in U.S. in the setting of a harm reduction for heroin addicts. It's not as popular for pain relief because metabolites (breakdown products) of methadone are also active and sedating. The medication tends to accumulate over time and prescribing it is trickier than writing a script for OxyContin.

Under Drug Enforcement Agency rules, methadone may be prescribed to people with opioid dependence so long as they are engaged in an ongoing psychiatric & recovery program. These are known as methadone clinics. Sadly, emotional connection and personal responsibility aren't as much emphasized in a typical methadone clinic. I know there are good ones, but there are not-so-good ones too.

Most customers only turn up for their daily dose, skipping optional life skills and vocational training. It's a shame really. Instead of regarding methadone harm reduction as a bridge to abstinence, an alarmingly high percentage of methadone customers are parked there indefinitely. You can say methadone is better than a cycle of typical chronic heroin dependency in this country, but I still don't believe anyone was born opioid-deficient. My problem with chronic methadone clinics is the trained helplessness they foster. And should you decide to quit methadone after a while on it, *mama mía* is that a tough and slow detox.

The harm-reduction philosophy (craving management with methadone), reduces petty crime and theft in the vicinity of the methadone clinic to the long-term detriment of the methadone customer. Now this philosophy is being applied more broadly with a newer pain medication with a unique chemical profile. The vanguard for opioid maintenance (harm reduction) is buprenorphine (Subutex®). More and more this is prescribed by general physicians to their opioid dependent patients.

Whether opiates or opioids, if you have taken them over a long enough period of time and in sufficient enough doses, the brain and nervous system will become adapted to these chemicals the same it does with alcohol. The mechanism of opiate dependence is not precisely the same, because the receptor is not the alcohol receptor but the *mu* opiate receptor, but tolerance happens with opioids as well as with alcohol.

Opiates are some of the most wildly prescribed drugs in America, and illicit opiates such as morphine or synthetic fentanyl analogues break records it seems year after year. In Sam Quinones' excellent book *Dreamland*, he traces two enterprising brothers from Mexico who studied prescribing patterns of American doctors. With their resulting analysis, they set up heroin distribution sites with a customer service model copying Domino's 30-minute Pizza delivery. The smart Mexican entrepreneurs franchised to cities where the largest number of OxyContin prescriptions were written. They wisely figured people would soon be in search of a cheaper commodity than OxyContin (in some places over $1 a milligram!) to soothe their opioid aches.

Like alcohol, opiates induce tolerance and physical dependence. As the level of drug increases remember the nervous system adapts by becoming less sensitive to the opiates. Like alcohol, the amount that worked to start becomes not enough. Stop and you get the uncomfortable feelings of withdrawal. These can include nausea, diarrhea, body aches, and generally feeling the *opposite* of blissful. Some describe withdrawal as feeling like you're trapped.

The best account of physical discomfort I heard of pertaining to opiate detox was from one of my patients. He was sweating a lot, feeling pretty bad. Mind you, he was detoxing from around fifteen times the dose of methadone you'd get in a methadone clinic. This was the toughest opioid case I've ever done and he was determined to get to zero. He had physiological withdrawal and sweating was one of his most bothersome symptoms. Colorfully, he described each drop of perspiration as, "coming out attached to a thorn." I can feel what he felt just writing about it.

Opiate withdrawal is usually not as dangerous as alcohol or sedative (benzo) detox. You might experience vomiting or diarrhea, both of which can lead to dehydration and electrolyte imbalances. The physical discomfort and suffering are severe, but almost never fatal. The main risk is quitting partway through detox. Tolerance levels reset lower; they might relapse back to the quantity/dose of opiates they used long before weaning. Because of tolerance, the body becomes more adapted and used to the presence of high levels of opiates.

As a person goes through withdrawal, this process happens in reverse and they become more sensitive to opiates. It's unfortunately common for someone who relapses to make a mental calculation, accounting for tolerance, and take <u>only half</u> of the dose they were taking before. Their tolerance level may have gone down tenfold. That is, they need ten times as much opiates right before starting detox, as when they started to get high the first time. If a person goes back to <u>half</u> the level that it took to get them high, if they're 10X more sensitive now, this could be far too much and lead to overdose.

Another risk with buying opiates from the street: you're never exactly sure what you get. It sounds macabre, but street dealers of opiates will frequently spike their product with very high levels of a synthetic fentanyl derivative for the specific purpose of *causing near deaths*. Epidemiologic studies in certain neighborhoods in New York and Philadelphia reveal clusters of O.D.s happen there about twice a year. This is, disgusting as it sounds, a branding flex for the drug dealers. People hear about the number of deaths from a specific brand or stamp mark on the envelope or baggy, and they want the same thing. They will be careful, right?

Marketing the drug by hospitalizing or accidentally killing some of the users appears to be the dealer's modus operandi. Sadly, there are always more customers to replace the victims and, for a time, demand increases. Opiate withdrawal feels horrible but as mentioned, aren't especially dangerous. Most of the habituated go through withdrawal "cold turkey." This expression comes from the bumps on the skin or standing up of the hairs that come along with opiate withdrawal, in medical language known as piloerection. Cold turkey kicking feels the worst.

Most people don't make it through because they relapse to using the drug again, but in most cases, home detox is safe. As always, nothing in here is specific medical advice, but if you can handle the suffering, most people come through opiate withdrawal just fine. When I finally stopped injectable opiates, I did it without any chemical help. Detox was the worst physical and emotional pain I've ever experienced. My tolerance levels were so high and my daily dose so astronomical, that my detox/withdrawal was super painful. Also, because of the high levels, I needed a long time to get my neurons working normally again.

During acute detox, I felt alternately hot and cold; a fever for an hour followed by freezing for forty-five minutes; now repeat. This temperature instability is not real, but it sure feels real. The body's temperature doesn't go through wild swings, but the part of the brain that manages temperature regulation (hypothalamus) is getting bad information as the neurons wake up from their opiate slumber. The sensation of being hot or cold is real, but the temperature fluctuations are not. I would sit in hot bath in order to deal with the freezing chills. In two minutes, I would be sweating again and on fire. I'd stand up out of the bath and let the cool air hit me until I was freezing cold again. Basically, hell.

Muscle aches, trouble sleeping, nausea, and diarrhea are also common with opiate withdrawal; I had all of these symptoms. Two other interesting things are runny nose and yawning. It's also par for the course to sweat a bit all the time, regardless of whether you feel hot or cold.

Overall, though, I have to say that opiate withdrawal is probably one of the safest detoxes there is. It is extremely rare for anyone who is otherwise physically healthy to have any significant medical problems from the withdrawal itself. Yes, it's uncomfortable, and the nausea and vomiting and diarrhea can lead to dehydration. This doesn't eliminate the suggestion that you involve a medical professional. But if you are worried about the withdrawal symptoms being so bad that you can't handle them physically or that something bad will happen to you, I would encourage you to proceed with medical guidance and let your doctor help you quit, because it's really not that bad (as long as you don't "pick up" again.

The level of opiates I was on when I finally stopped was absurdly high. I won't recount the details here, but suffice it to say, I haven't met anyone who was on *more than me* in terms of morphine equivalence (the standard use to compare opiates to opiates). If I can get through it, you can get through it.

As long as you don't have contraindications to taking these over-the-counter medications, ibuprofen and Tylenol can help reduce muscle aches and pains. Melatonin is helpful for sleep, as is valerian root. Immodium (loperamide) really can be helpful if you have diarrhea from stopping opioids.

And a visit with you physician for baclofen for more significant detox aches, Zofran for nausea and maybe even a few days of a sleeping medication can be valuable tools for getting you to zero. We spoke of buprenorphine/Suboxone® for maintenance–which I don't recommend in general–but a short course of it can be helpful. These medications must be prescribed by a licensed prescriber, but I find them helpful to make opioid detox more comfortable.

The main key is your attitude. If you're committed to change, and you promise yourself you'll do everything to keep moving forward, detox won't be nearly as difficult as for someone who resists.

–13–
MARIJUANA DETOX

A 52-year-old man undergoes treatment for cancer. His tumors shrink, but a side effect of the treatment is poor appetite. He looks on the Internet and discovers others have used "Mary-Jane" to improve their appetite. Industrious, he buys some from a local dispensary selling newly legal THC.

The following day, our man is in the emergency room, confused, disoriented and muttering. Repeat scans show the tumors are unchanged, stable. His wife shows the ER doctor a mostly-consumed syringe of liquid marijuana extract. It has over 330 mg of THC, the psychoactive ingredient in marijuana. Our man has gotten so high, he doesn't know where–or who– he is. After a couple of days in a hospital room, he's back to normal.

It's unfortunately an urban myth that nobody ever died because of marijuana. This is simply not true. There is also a well characterized withdrawal symptom profile. Regular marijuana use produces a habit use pattern just like any of the other substances we've covered in this book. Once people become habitual users of the drug, the same adaptation of brain communication processes in the neurons covered earlier happens with weed too. Because people don't have a severe physical withdrawal pattern, like from alcohol, opiates or sedatives, it doesn't mean there isn't significant *psychological* withdrawal.

To understand marijuana detox, let's take a closer look at what happens with marijuana intoxication. Marijuana is a cannabinoid, and it works at the anandamide receptor. The anandamide receptor is named for the Sanskrit word for bliss. The bliss you feel with marijuana is characterized by *relaxed interest*. The most active moment of the endocannabinoid system – not from pot – is right after you're born. A few minutes after birth, the most important activities for a newborn are bonding with mother and getting fed. One well-known effect of marijuana increased appetite. Augmented hunger from THC was the mechanism used to treat our man when cancer sapped his appetite.

Peak natural endocannabinoid surge plays a role nursing success and for the empathetic connection made from baby to mother *by producing a state of relaxed interest*. The new mom feels a rush of trust and satisfaction due to oxytocin, and the bonding so vital for the survival of our species starts of on the right foot. Oxytocin (hormone) also helps with uterine shrinking and vascular contraction so her anatomy can get back to normal and bleeding can cease. Which brings up an interesting aspect of all the substances humans use habitually: they're bio-hacks of an existing signal system. Whether bliss (opioids), relaxed interest (cannabis), elation and heightened focus (cocaine) or others we use chemicals to exploit existing neurobiology.

When ingest the active ingredients in marijuana, we activate the endocannabinoid system (anandamide). This stimulates food consumption, and it helps even the most boring events seem more interesting. Marijuana provides relief from the drudgery of day-to-day life, but when used over long period of time, neuroadaptation occurs as does with all substances. Demotivation and apathetic dissipation of life's energies are also hallmarks of long-term use.

The Cannabis Withdrawal Syndrome (CWS) includes restless boredom, sleeplessness, mood swings and frustration. There's no nausea or diarrhea, and physical symptoms, loss of appetite and symptoms mimicking depression are common for two to four weeks following cessation in daily users.

There are no replacement drugs for marijuana; the best practice is to just ride it out. In a month life will seem interesting again, and food will start to taste good. Most of the problem with marijuana dependence has to do with the social and cultural uses. Although some people ingest or smoke marijuana solo, it's frequently shared socially or used as an adjunct to sexual intercourse. Acclimating to social interactions without the mind-altering drug can be a challenge. Many of my patients were anxious when they thought about sex with their partners without taking anything. I may sound like a broken record here, but at that risk I'll say it again: exercise is very helpful.

In fact, for all of the substance habits, exercise is a wonderful antidote to most symptoms of withdrawal. Sleep disturbance is quite common following abstinence or reduction in drug use, both for neurochemical and habit reasons. Exercise makes the body physically tired, which helps a lot at bedtime. Exercise is also a natural antidepressant, as is sunshine, and spending time outdoors. While it is probably the last thing you want to hear while kicking dope, taking a walk if you can is one of the best things for you.

To better understand the value of exercise, let's go back to the model of brain evolution. When we first crawled out of the ooze and began running on land millions of years ago, chasing and avoiding being caught were paramount. Key to survival, whether as hunter or prey, was the ability to move about, locomotion. Our brains haven't changed, except how little activity is required in modern times to feed and shelter ourselves.

The brain-body dichotomy is false: they are not separate entities. Though when we feel tired, the sensation is in our body, "fatigue" is not actually located in the body. It is just what our brains tell us: an organizing system. Exercise is savored by the brain, it is salient, and essential–always. Activity also brings vital oxygen, removes carbon dioxide, increases blood flow to the far corners, and stokes calorie burn. Movement makes us more alert and more rested after. How can you beat that?

I've mentioned that activity is an anti-depressant; a fact supported by research. Check out what Drs. Craft & Perna had to say about it in their overview of exercise as treatment for depression in *Prim Care Companion J Clin Psychiatry*. (2004; 6(3): 104–111):

Research also suggests that the benefits of exercise involvement may be long lasting. Depressed adults who took part in a fitness program displayed significantly *greater improvements in depression, anxiety, and self-concept than those in a control group after 12 weeks of training (BDI reduction of 5.1 [fitness program] vs. 0.9 [control], p < .001). The exercise participants also maintained many of these gains through the 12-month follow-up period.*

People who are active are less depressed. I remember after my own fentanyl detox sitting in our small apartment in Sacramento. I was feeling sorry for myself about the mess I had made of my life, my then girlfriend (Hello Dr./Mrs. Giles) said the meanest thing ever spoken by one human being to another:

"Why don't you go outside and take a walk?"

I was shocked, furious and more than a little scared. Near rock-bottom, I had retreated so far into my apartment–cave, I feared going outside. Contemplating a walk around the block was itself overwhelming. Gripped in paralyzing fear, I had to prove I wasn't scared. I gingerly inched down the front steps. The afternoon sun dappled the sidewalk. Nobody was around so I set a bold checkpoint: the mailbox at the corner. I made it, and hustled back inside.

I couldn't make it around the block the first time. With great effort, the mailbox was nearly too much. The next morning, I walked halfway around the block to the alley. On day three, I made it all the way around the block. Of course, she was right and I was in a sad habit of thinking myself as helpless. A hallmark of the chronically depressed. I didn't realize that I'd sold myself short regarding the challenges I could handle. Besides depression, helplessness is a common finding in late-stage substance habit dependence.

While tolerance increases with drug use, intolerance of reality worsens. When we're wedded to substances as a source of escape, life itself feels too much to bear, and progressively tougher the less we face it and deal. Sometimes even standing in line at the grocery store becomes an unbearable task. Maybe we explode at one of the people in line. We count eleven items in her cart but the line is for ten items or fewer. Supermarket police.

Tolerance and intolerance are two facets of substance habit/recovery. As we gain freedom and become less dependent on addictive cyclic behaviors, we're able to do more: our lives expand. Our happiness is directly proportional to tolerance of uncertainty.

If we are okay with work-in-progress selves and can "roll with it" as they say, then everything bothers us less. When life is a bitch, we want more drugs to ease the unfair suffering we all feel. Drugs give is the illusion of power over our circumstances. In a perverse way, the substances keep us crippled even though we take them in order to feel stronger and to have less pain.

Exercise refocuses the mind. No matter how badly we feel about ourselves, getting out of the house for some fresh air, going to the gym, or even doing a few pushups in the living room are acts of defiance toward our negative self-talk. No matter what we think about ourselves and our situation, we can leap over that, sometimes literally. We act our way into feeling better.

So, why don't you do yourself a favor right now, and stand up where you are if you're sitting and stretch. If you're listening to this as an audio book or driving, then wait until it is safe for you to do so. But when you get to your next stop, stretch a bit. Just be aware of your body. If your doctor wouldn't mind, get a little exercise. I promise it will change your frame of mind.

And the most important part of ditching a THC habit is not to dabble. Just leave it all behind. It's not that strong of a withdrawal symptom set, the real hook, much like with cigarettes (tobacco), is the habit. I spoke with a patient this week who gave up meth smoking but replaced it with marijuana. Most would agree: a person with a marijuana problem is better off than a person dependent on methamphetamine to get by. But the usual course in a situation like this one is to drift back to smoking pot.

If something is easy to quit, it's also easy to pick back up in a few weeks later on when pressures come again to plague you. Marijuana reduces our motivation and saps our drive. And if you read Gregory Berent's unsettling book called Tell Your Children, you might come away with some downright fear about continuing to use THC.

The concentrations available commercially and at dispensaries should give anyone pause, because they're strong enough to radically alter behavior: even to the point of homicide.

–14–
SEDATIVES/BENZODIAZEPINES AND DETOX

Benzodiazepines are among the most commonly prescribed drugs in America. They are given for sleep, anxiety, panic, seizures, and rarely muscle problems. In a 2019 review of prescribing patterns in the U.S., published in the distinguished *Journal of the American Medical Association*, Drs. Agarwal and Landon found nearly 8% of all ambulatory visits to general practice clinics sent patients out with a prescription for a "benzo."

They also reported the rate of benzo prescriptions had doubled over the past two decades, from 3.4% to 7.4% between 2003 and 2015 (though psychiatrists held steady at only ~30% of their visits over the same time resulting in a prescription for something like Valium®). So many benzos were prescribed for anxiety in the State of New York, that their DEA reclassified them to require a special prescription, and to be filled for no more than five days at a time.

Also alarming, the death rate per 100,000 people due to drugs like Xanax®, or Ativan®, skyrocketed from less than one (0.6) to over four (4.4). Elderly people made up the bulk of the excess mortality figures, but younger folks were not spared. Why the increase in prescriptions for benzos, such as Klonopin®? Why the allure and why are they so habit forming? Let's dig the biology of benzodiazepines, why they're so hard to stop, and how to ditch them if you've decided it's time. tl; dr – slowly.

Benzodiazepines work at yet a different receptor in your nervous system: GABA. This acronym is shorthand for *gamma amino butyric acid*–you see why we say GABA. It's a naturally occurring neurotransmitter that balances dopamine and others. I think about this molecule as the "brake" on our thoughts. Elevated GABA levels floating past your nerve endings make them less likely to fire. The feeling of elevated GABA is one of calm, or relaxed fuzziness.

Benzodiazepine receptors are part of the GABA receptor complex on neurons, and their activation causes a similar effect as does alcohol or opiates. The effect is to make the cell more resistant to stimulation. Said more simply, they are sedatives or "downers." Benzos reduce overall activity in neurons. Makes sense that they're prescribed for anxiety, yes?

Anxiety can feel like racing thoughts. Benzos will cause you to have fewer thoughts, which might be helpful if too many of your thoughts are scary or unsettling. In cases of acute severe anxiety, benzodiazepines can be life-saving. They are still frequently prescribed following bouts of major grief (i.e. the loss of a child), but benzos, as you can tell, have a dark side. As with all bio-active substances, including psychiatric medicines of every stripe, the brain becomes adapted to the presence of the chemical. Tolerance applies here too.

By now, you can guess if the response is sedation, then the adaptation is anxiety or enhanced neuronal transmission. The nerves are used to being muffled, so they turn up the amplifier. They dial up sensitivity settings by increasing the number of receptors, as well as making other changes inside of the nerve cell.

Benzodiazepines work to cause sedation by opening a door in of the cell called the chloride channel. Through it flows chloride ions and when enough pass through, this changes the electrical charge on the neuron. The changed surface charge makes it more resistant to stimulation.

Benzodiazepines are metabolized by the liver, and when their blood levels fall, the neurons miss their sedating effects. The withdrawal symptoms associated with benzodiazepines, dreadfully, are indistinguishable from the *original condition that prompted their use*. This is one of the worst aspects of benzos. It's also how they're very different from alcohol or opiates during withdrawal. When we withdraw from opiates, there is a distinct syndrome of opiate withdrawal. People "kicking" heroin or similar drugs (e.g. OxyContin, Vicodin) have an unmistakable sensation of opiate withdrawal.

There is suffering and a feeling of helplessness when withdrawing from opioids, but the physical discomfort isn't exactly simple physical pain. There are aches and general intolerance for physical touch, but runny nose, yawning, and diarrhea are not the *reasons why people take opiates*. The withdrawal symptoms are different from the feeling you had before you started, these drugs.

Anxiety, stress or trouble sleeping are the main reasons why people take benzodiazepines. When withdrawing from them, the symptoms are primarily anxiety, fear, sleeplessness and dread. Free-floating terror or fear doesn't *feel like* it is a withdrawal syndrome from the drug. You just feel scared. Users start Valium and drugs like it, because they're anxious and scared. Perhaps they're scared because they have avoided dealing with life as it comes. Maybe they had trouble sleeping and developed a habit dependency. But when they come off benzos, they feel frightened.

The amount of time it takes to come off of drugs like Valium depends on a number of factors. Principal among them is how long a person has been using these drugs. If you've been on them for only a few days or a couple of weeks, then the chances are your withdrawal symptoms will be pretty mild. But after a few months or years, stopping will almost certainly produce a lot of apprehension and dread.

There's also the risk of seizure. With high doses, and/or long-standing benzo use, the brain becomes very adapted. If you take your foot off the brake (sedatives), then the revved-up brain cells (neurons) can sometimes generalize into a seizure. For this reason, it is strongly advised that you take benzodiazepine withdrawal seriously. It's more dangerous than quitting an opiate habit. This is due in part because of seizures, but also for those with weak cardiovascular systems, blood pressure and heart rate elevations can cause trouble.

Also, the deep sense of fear/anxiety that can result from benzodiazepine withdrawal, not to mention sleeplessness, should be dealt with carefully. The point is generally to reach abstinence. The goal is to not need sedatives or sleeping pills in order to sleep. It is better to take things slowly. Please involve a doctor, because it is important to carefully wean off of these drugs.

Assuming that you're in the group that has been on benzos for a long time, then a slow progressive regimen of reducing the dose week to week is likely the best plan. As you go, you'll tend to feel a bit anxious. The withdrawal is relatively predictable, and switching to a longer-acting sedative or benzodiazepine can smooth your transition. We want to avoid the peaks and valleys—over sedation or over anxiousness—that go with the shorter-acting drugs. Remember, all the sedatives are synergistic with each other, and alcohol should be avoided if you are taking a drug like a benzodiazepine.

I'll restate the importance of exercise here, as there are a few things that are as helpful for benzodiazepine withdrawal. An exercised body (physically tired) cues the circadian brain that it's time for sleep. Don't skip the workout. Additionally, there are other drugs in the anti-seizure class that can be helpful. One of the ones I prescribe most commonly for benzodiazepine withdrawal is gabapentin (see the 'gaba' in there?). There are a few cautions, but in general I find most people have a better time coming off drugs such as Xanax and Valium if they use Neurontin. See your doctor.

Gabapentin is not addictive. You cannot get high on gabapentin, but it reduces neuronal transmission via the GABA receptor complex. This works similar to benzodiazepines but without the high. It can provide just enough "brake" to reduce some of the terror and physical anxiety that goes along with benzodiazepine withdrawal. Ask your doctor about gabapentin or other drugs in the same anti-seizure family; they may help. Using them increases the margin of safety away from seizure too.

One of the trickiest aspects of benzodiazepine withdrawal is the long-term re-wiring, or restoration, of the receptors. By now you're very familiar with this process. It is normal and what most people mean when they say detox. Assuming this goes well for you, and if you have a doctor helping you, then at some point you'll get down to zero.

But even at zero the brain has not finished recuperating. It takes time for brain reorganization. I think of it like moving into a new house. When you first arrive, you've got all of your stuff in boxes and it has to be put away. Not all of the unpacking can happen simultaneously, so some boxes have to go in some rooms and wait until other ones are opened. The same sort of thing is happening inside the brain.

The brain adapts to the presence of substances by changing the number and sensitivity of receptors on its cells. Habitual exposure causes more permanent cell adaptations. Discontinuing substances (detox), forces the brain to adapt again. With millions of little remodeling projects (each synapse where the drug used to have an effect) they can't be completed all at once. Reset takes time, and there is probably an order of priority as well. Ultra-rapid detox for opiates has been tried, but simply removing the substance isn't enough to quickly restore normal function.

Detox from benzos has a lot of ups and downs. The clinical course, or how crappy you feel, is more or less gradual improvement over time. From month to month, you will feel much better leaving the drugs behind. If we graphed "how you feel" over time and zoomed out to the "month view" the line would go upward nicely toward 'happy'. Zooming in to the day or hour, and the same graph would look jagged. Since we're near-term creatures, especially when stressed, it's easy to give up and relapse following a string of rough days. But don't quit the process. All substance habits take time to form and more time to replace.

With just your own mind as the measurement device of your detox progress, it's hard to see the improvement you've made. Humans jump to conclusions; that is the nature of being a pattern-forming creature. Here's a reminder: how you feel on any one day is only a tiny piece of your recovery arc. If you kept track, you would see that jagged mood improvement line slopes up toward *better*. Steady, by jerks.

One of my favorite stories about a benzodiazepine patient is a woman who came in to a treatment center here in Malibu. She was eighty-one years old and had been intervened upon by her two adult sons. They told me their mother was acting wild, running around her yard in the nude, and screaming at the neighbors. She reluctantly agreed to a thirty-day treatment program. She denied all of their assertions and did it only to get her boys off her back.

Despite the three-star chef, equine therapy (pet the horsey), and on-call massages, she refused to participate in the program whatsoever. She wouldn't go to group, or even talk to the counselors. Total stonewall. Weirdly, from my perspective, she displayed *no evidence of benzodiazepine withdrawal.* The bizarre behavior described by her boys sounded more like alcohol abuse than benzos. She said she took Valium "from time to time," but she didn't have to. I didn't order any for her and she didn't seem to mind. She refused to provide a drug test, of course.

For three weeks, and she was pack-mule stubborn. As discharge day approached, she began to report a few concerns. She had an upset stomach and trouble sleeping. Since this is one of those frou-frou addiction treatment centers, a holistic herbalist was brought in. He had nothing concrete to offer, and her symptoms slowly worsened. In the last days of her treatment, she was sweating, frightened, and had huge dilated pupils. In a private moment, she admitted she was in withdrawal from Valium. It had taken almost a month for her liver to process the massive store of benzodiazepines in her body.

She told me she tried to quit several times over the years, but she never got past this point. I learned, her husband was a doctor, and one of the first in America to prescribe Valium back in the 1960s. Remember "Mother's Little Helper," the Rolling Stones song? Long hours at work may have strained their relationship. The doc brought home a new drug, and she tried some samples. He found her much calmer as a result. She didn't mind so much that he was gone all day, leaving her with tussling young boys. He kept her on the drug–samples for the next forty years.

She found a new source after her husband died. She was on a staggering amount of Valium, especially for an octogenarian. She was taking so much, and her metabolism of it was so slow, that she needed weeks to process her internal stockpile.

She must have felt crummy along the way, but because of a combination of determination and general stubbornness, she was able to tough out her symptoms early on. As she got lower and lower in her body's overall remaining sequester, she began to have classic benzodiazepine withdrawal symptoms.

She and I had a decision to make together. If someone is on benzodiazepines for a few weeks, I recommend coming off, naturally. But she had had an extremely high dose for a very long time, and she was much nearer the end of her life than the beginning. I talked to her about the role of the drug and the risks of taking too much and "acting crazy." She understood what I was getting at, and promised to try and be more modest in her yard.

She recognized that her boys were worried about her and were trying to take care of their mom, not controlling her—so long as she was able to control herself. She admitted to periods of sadness and moodiness, especially since the death of her husband. She missed him. Despite the questionable management of his wife's feelings, she was very fond of him and was, in many ways, staying connected to him by taking the drug he prescribed for her. She was emotionally bonded to the drug as much as she was physically dependent on it.

Meeting together with her sons, we all decided that the better part of valor was for her to remain on Valium from there on out. It was certainly treating her anxiety, if only because decades of use made her permanently anxious. Now she didn't have to hide it or be secretive. Her sons knew what was happening, and they knew what to look for. Their relationships immediately improved and she went on to live for many more years.

In summary, benzodiazepines are tricky to come off of, especially if other substance habits are present too. Their main withdrawal symptom is anxiety, and too-fast withdrawal (like alcohol) can lead to seizure. It's best to ween slowly under the guidance and care of a physician.

–15–
Z-DRUGS AND DETOX

Some pills marketed as sleep aids are not technically benzodiazepines, but they act much the same way once they're swallowed. Though not chemically identical, they have a similar effect as Valium. In 2017, zolpidem was the 50th most commonly prescribed medication in the United States, with more than 15 million prescriptions. Granted FDA approval in 1992 for short-term treatment of insomnia, nonbenzodiazepines are now the most prescribed sedative in America. Many of the "Z-drugs," named for zolpidem, the granddaddy, were touted as non-addictive because their effect would be gone by sunrise.

Thus, a marketing angle was born for a drug called Ambien. The trade name is a play on words: 'am' for morning, and bien, like the Spanish word for 'well'. It's like saying good morning. The sales message is take it, get to sleep, and be fresh by morning. What a marvel medicine has wrought! Only benefits and *no side effects*. Whenever you hear that, be suspicious. Every medication affects physiology. There are always side effects no matter the substance. With a drug that works like a short-acting Valium, you know there are bound to be problems.

In the case of Ambien (zolpidem, generic) the drug performs like a benzodiazepine. The chemical structure is different, but the net effect at the neurons is extremely similar. These drugs open chloride channels that dampen nerve transmission, just like alcohol or other sedatives.

A NYT article from 2006 highlighted the increasing concern over the Z-drugs. The reporter covered a research paper which was presented at the American Academy of Forensic Sciences. They looked at the effects of Ambien on motorists:

"…drivers who took Ambien were more likely to run into stationary objects like light poles or parked vehicles than drivers who had consumed drugs or alcohol, and were more likely to be oblivious to arresting officers."

The author of the study called many of these incidents "just extremely bizarre." The warnings required by the Food and Drug Administration for Ambien's label say that it can cause sleepwalking and hallucinations in some cases, and cautions against combining it with alcohol.

That same year, Congressman Patrick J. Kennedy was on Ambien and cough syrup (Phenergan) when he was cited by D.C. police on Capitol Hill. Though Kennedy drove in the wrong lane until he smashed into a barrier, he had no recollection of the incident. He didn't even remember getting out of bed, only that he was late for a vote on an important bill. He was basically sleep-driving. Kennedy later sought treatment for his substance habits and returned to congress.

Z drugs are more likely to impair memory and recall. They affect short-term to long-term memory transfer, but their after-effects may improve sports performance. Michael Phelps admitted he used Ambien to get to sleep during his swimming career. The men's 2012 Australian Olympic relay team used Stilnox (Ambien) together the night before their medal round, to some controversy. Z-drug use was widespread at the London Olympics, the decreased anxiety, and better sleep improved performance.

Ambien reminds me of an interesting story. Once I treated a 30-ish, petite woman for an Ambien habit. A super achiever attorney in intellectual property law, she started taking the drug in law school in order to sleep. I.P. is a complex area of law, and her firm handled the biggest cases. She was working her way toward partner under tremendous pressure.

Insomnia returned, and she got a prescription from her doctor. He gave her a short course of Ambien, ten milligrams, with standard recommendations to get some exercise and to pursue a better work-life balance. She found immediate relief at bedtime, sleeping the night through for the first time in years. Ambien was her salvation. Because she was able to sleep, she was able to work more.

Unfortunately, because she was able to work more, she soon slept less. As with the Olympic swimmers, she wanted to achieve more. She felt the drug enhanced her creativity, that it was her ally and her secret weapon.

She started with ten milligrams a day, and that was soon doubled. Over the years, she escalated her dose, a classic case of tolerance. She doubled her dose again. Ultimately had to go beyond medical practice, to street dealers, in order to find her supply. She had plenty of money, and with an essentially unlimited supply of Ambien, her dose continued to climb.

She took Ambien throughout the day but her work suffered. Once, while she was in a conference negotiating a big settlement deal between two major technology companies, she lost her mind. She started talking in gibberish, stared out the window for twenty minutes, in an unresponsive daze. Then she snapped. She grabbed a tall stack of papers and threw it at the CEO of one of the two companies. When the other one laughed, she screamed at him. This kind of display did not endear her to her bosses. But they recognized something must be wrong with their wonder girl.

By the time she got to treatment, she had increased her daily pill take from one to two to *sixty*. No joke–she was taking on average *sixty ten-milligram Ambien pills per day*. You can't imagine the psychiatric effects on this poor young woman.

She was open to help from the start. Beaten by Ambien, and she was willing to learn better how to handle stress. As we talked over the next few days, it became clear to her she did not enjoy her job. She was overdoing work and win the approbation of her father. He was a very successful attorney, but she didn't even like law. She originally studied biology, and that's where her heart lay. Underneath the tough exterior, she craved acceptance and love. She did what many with substance habits do–stay and leave at the same time. Stay physically, leave mentally.

A top performer at the law firm, she was incredibly high-functioning due to her work ethic, intelligence, and drive. But she would check out emotionally because she was in the wrong job *for her*.

When she realized the substances were a buffer against her feelings, she ditched Ambien forever. Her detox was impossibly fast *and* smooth. Ambien is short-acting, but she had been on it around the clock years, and at impossibly high doses.

Ordinarily, the Z drugs, take time to come off. Sleep disturbance is the most significant complaint and rebound insomnia is nearly universal, but for her she was off completely in a couple of weeks. She took up tennis again, a sport she played in college. She challenged everyone to singles or doubles on the court. She channeled her energy into exercise, and as if something had been unlocked, she was very forthcoming about her fears and anxieties.

Within two weeks, she no longer needed any benzodiazepine support. She stayed on Neurontin for a couple more weeks, but she even quit that. She never had a seizure, and she was able to speak openly with her father and repair their relationship. Last I heard, she was married with her second child on the way.

It's hard to explain how someone could be on near-lethal daily doses of Ambien, and detox that quickly. But over the years of helping people quit, I've seen the most important element of drug and alcohol withdrawal is the person's state of mind. Let me explain.

If you attempt detox, but plan to use substances again to manage your feelings–in other words, you're not here for the long haul–then detox is agony. Every single muscle ache and every lost moment of sleep during withdrawal and detox feels pointless. If in the back of your mind you plan to go back to using or drinking. Your mind will torment you. Needless suffering.

But if your life has deteriorated to the point where you can see drugs and alcohol are worn out solutions, that they cause more mischief than help, then detox is an entirely different experience. Perhaps the physiology is no different, but how we feel about ourselves in relation to the world makes all the difference in the course (and tempo) of withdrawal.

If you are *done*, and by that, I mean that you're not going to live your life under the lash of alcohol or drugs, then you'll probably find detox and withdrawal remarkably easy. The final time may be the easiest you've ever had. This was my experience at the end, but not along the way when I hadn't made the commitment to stop.

I was taking an incredibly high dose of daily injectable opioids, and I was off it within a few days. Yes, I felt agony, the bathtub detox was hard, but I had made a decision I wasn't going to do this anymore. My commitment afforded a quantum of grace.

As I went through fentanyl withdrawal, I didn't know what was next for me professionally or personally. I feared a person like me couldn't be helped, that I was doomed. Nevertheless, I persisted. I made a decision to stay sober "one day at a time," no matter what. The outcome was not my responsibility, the effort was.

"One day at a time, but beginning tomorrow" is probably the greatest substance habit maintenance strategy of all time. I'll use drugs today, but tomorrow everything will be different. This is the way that we make a deal with ourselves that we don't have to change. When tomorrow comes, we keep using the substances, or drinking, or whatever the addiction is, because we can always say that tomorrow I'll quit. Addicts and alcoholics and others caught in a substance habit loop are notorious for wanting *credit for their intentions*.

I knew that this was between me and the Universe. There was no one else I was getting sober for. I was choosing to see what was on the other side of this problem. The adventure had come full circle, and no matter what came next, I wasn't going back to my old way of life.

Despite nausea, sweating, and feeling crappy, I had a sparkling gem of hope. I knew my life was going to change. Taken from this perspective, a runny nose, loose bowels and back pain were the price of admission for a new life. I didn't mind nearly as much as I had in the past. Looking back, it is hard to believe how easy it was for me to detox.

So, you can think of the Z-drugs just like benzodiazepines. They work about the same and their detox is similar. The key with this detox is to get help and guidance from a good doctor. Medicines like gabapentin are helpful and insomnia can, and should, be managed with non-pharmacologic strategies.

16 AMPHETAMINES, OTHER STIMULANTS AND DETOX

60,000 years ago, in a cave at Shanidar (on today's map Iraq), a Neanderthal man was laid to rest surrounded by flowers. The plants tell the story how our relatives, *Homo neanderthalensis*, used plants as food, medicine, and for ceremony. Included in the flora were pollen grains from the herbal stimulant ephedra.

Stimulants, like ephedra, coca, and paan were used by man long before recorded history. Around 850 AD, an Ethiopian goat herder observed his goats leaping and dancing after they ate the berries of a new bush. They were too bitter for him to eat, so he mashed them up in water and boiled a brew. As the legend goes, the effects were delightful, allowing him to complete his morning prayers in no time.

Anyone who's had a cup of coffee or strong tea has experienced a stimulant, particularly its mood and energy elevating effects. Stimulants can get much stronger. They increase our ability to focus, sociability, and energy. They can also be abused and become a habit, which is the subject of this chapter.

Commonly troublesome stimulants include amphetamines, cocaine, MDMA (ecstasy), nicotine, and cocaine. Much milder than cocaine, the areca nut is chewed throughout Asia for its stimulant effect. Its stimulant compounds don't cause bizarre behavior like meth does, but betel nut chewers get mouth cancer and along the way a ghastly amount of red saliva. Indirectly betel nut chewing causes morbidity and death, just not as expediently as cocaine.

Cocaine's effects were first described formally in a paper by Sigmund Freud. The Viennese doctor gave it out to cheer up his depressed patients, and it temporarily worked. He may have developed a problem with it himself, we know he described his tongue going numb when he ingested the drug.

Freud's frozen tongue report caught the attention of a young New York doctor named William Halsted. The Bellevue surgeon was interested in using the new drug from Germany for surgical pain control. He thought if he could inject some of this cocaine along the course of a nerve, he could make the area felt by that nerve go numb too. If it didn't have feeling or pain, then he could operate freely on a patient's arm or leg.

Dr. Halsted was an ambitious researcher, but he didn't have a suitable human subject that he could test his anatomic theory of anesthesia upon. He made *himself* the study subject, and mapped the course of the superficial nerves in his arms and legs by injecting his arms and legs with the drug. The nerve blocks that he devised are still used today for surgery. I used to give lidocaine for the very same blocks in my patients. Unfortunately, Dr. Halsted became habituated to the cocaine. His use escalated, with regular shipments of the drug from Germany, until finally even he couldn't get an adequate supply. Dr. Halstead missed a lot of work, was progressively more agitated, and despite being a brilliant surgeon, his practice fell apart.

Morphine gives totally different effect. A sedative instead of a stimulant, but it must have worked well enough. Here lies a curious aspect of drug addiction. Halsted remained on morphine even after he left New York and transferred to Johns Hopkins in Baltimore. As far as we know, he remained on morphine the rest of his life—but he never went back to cocaine.

Stimulants work in the brain by increasing and speeding nerve transmission. Opposite to the effect of a sedative, stimulants make neurons twitchy and jumpy. There are many interesting technical details about how the receptors work. I encourage you to read further about them if you like, but they are beyond the scope of this book. Suffice it to say, if stimulants speed up nerves, you would logically conclude stimulant withdrawal symptoms are the mirror opposite. You'd be right. People kicking speed are tired, unfocused, lethargic, and have trouble staying awake.

Amphetamines are routinely prescribed for attention deficit and hyperactivity disorder, or ADHD. Millions of children are on stimulants. We don't yet know the extent to which these drugs affect the developing brain of a child. These are tough decisions for any family (ask your doctor). I approach them with a skeptical eye for long-term effects.

The presence of any drug while the brain is developing will have greater profound impact than it would on a mature brain. To that end, our brains continue to develop over our whole lives, which is why we always need to be careful with the drugs we take.

The withdrawal symptoms from uppers, as mentioned include fatigue, lethargy, and confusion. Depression is common in acute withdrawal, as is overeating. Stimulants decrease the appetite, so reliably that they're prescribed as weight-loss aides. The dangerous drug combination from the 1990s, Fen-Phen, is a combination of two stimulants. Sadly, many heart valves were damaged as a side effect of taking Fen-phen for weight loss.

I observed prodigious post-stimulant weight gain firsthand when I was in rehab. A pathologist detoxed from two years of methamphetamine abuse. He had a daily habit, and on admission he was cachectic, skeletal. But not for long. He exploited the excellent sustenance in the institution's cafeteria, piling high his plates at the buffet. The doctor was there for two months, and he gained about one pound per day. Sixty pounds heavier, he was overweight the day he was discharged from rehab.

Besides weight gain, a few days of fatigue, and feeling down for a while, kicking stimulants isn't that difficult from a physical/detox/withdrawal standpoint. The challenge is in breaking the habit routine. Stimulants make us feel powerful. Invincible. The can make tedious work seem compelling and interesting.

I helped a young methamphetamine user who worked as a "land man" down in Louisiana. In case you aren't familiar with that occupation, a land man performs title searches on real property. In case the owner strikes oil, the land man's detective work back to Spanish land grants will confirm the chain of ownership. You'd hate to strike oil and then have someone else come along and tell you the mineral rights weren't transferred in 1871, and therefore the oil belongs to someone else.

Poring over the records in the parish courthouse is about as tedious as a job gets. Ensuring the lot description covers precisely the parcel in the contract, traced back through history is enough to put anyone to sleep. Make a mistake and potentially millions are lost. That is, it's hard to focus without methamphetamine.

For the land man, the drug made him better and faster at his job. It was rough when he quit meth. Rummaging through old maps and records was too much to bear and he changed careers. He stayed in the energy sector, but as an investor instead of in his old job.

Two more quick stories about stimulants and then I'll let you go on to the opioid epidemic chapter. First, the Wehrmacht. After that, we'll talk about the myth of permanent brain damage from meth.

In 1943 Hitler was pretty screwed. Barbarossa had collapsed, and in a stunning reversal, the German 6th army was crushed at Stalingrad. America was fully in the war, and the Reich no longer ruled the skies. Germany was out first-round draft picks for her army, and increasingly she recruited teenagers and old WWI vets to fight for survival. But the crafty Fuhrer had a wonder-weapon up his sleeve: crystal meth.

35 million tablets of the potent stimulant, Pervitin (methamphetamine) would make his super soldiers *uber alles*. They had been on it during the blitz of France, what could go wrong? Again the Austrian miscalculated. Meth is a stimulant, and it *did* help the army stay awake longer. But it didn't turn them into super soldiers, and fortunately for freedom-loving people around the world, even Nazi soldiers need sleep.

Hitler himself had a speed habit (and an oxycodone habit). Maybe he thought his fighting forces should be more like their leader. But speed in the Wehrmacht was no match for allied commitment to end the Nazi scourge. Starving, undersupplied, surrounded, and fighting on the wrong side of morality, they had hallucinations and lost focus in battle.

And finally, let's take on the myth of permanent brain damage from methamphetamine. In what's become a classic image in the canon of addiction medicine, the colored images of the brain of an "addict" and a "normal" person were compared side by side. Even one month after stopping, the image showed permanent injury.

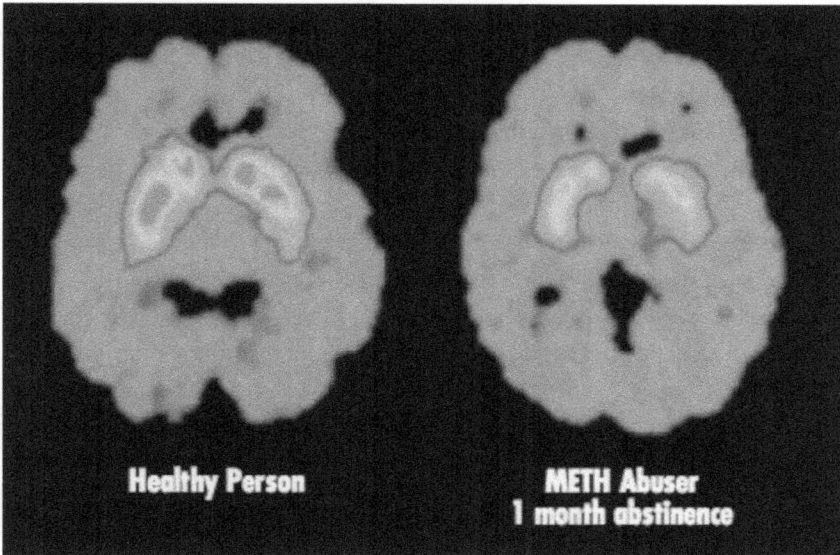

The former had dark, ominous looking dropouts/holes in the dopamine part of the brain. The normal brain was bright and colorful. The message: just say no.

I never liked that image. It always seemed too fatalistic to me, depressing. The brain is plastic and can recover from injury or stroke. Surely the magnificent brain could bounce back from methamphetamine injury, no?

I found a follow up image that didn't get as much attention. It shows the brain of a guy with a meth habit who stopped for 14 months. Cold turkey, totally abstinent. He simply gave up the habit of using meth and got back in the scanner.

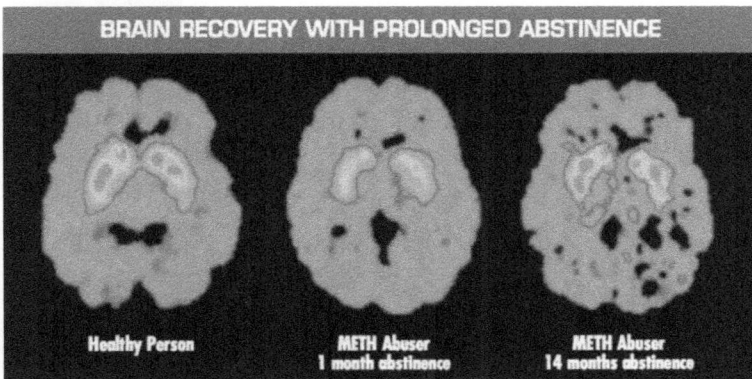

In this PET scan (a type of functional brain imaging) you can see for yourself the return of the healthy red color what was previously "damaged" by meth use. The brain is remarkably resilient. Be kind to it and you'll be delighted with how it repays you. Most importantly, even if you need to kick a stimulant habit like methamphetamine or cocaine, give yourself time, remember to exercise, eat well and know that everything's going to turn out better than you imagined.

Nutrition is critical in recovery from all substance habits, but especially so with stimulant use. The little packets of neurochemicals are over-activated by these stimulant chemicals and much of the "depression" experienced in early abstinence is due to low levels of thinking molecules.

They need to be rebuilt, and doing so takes time. The amino acid tyrosine is the precursor to dopamine, a key neurotransmitter. The issue of which foods to eat to restore adequate neurochemical supply and balance has not been fully studied. For now, if you want to ensure adequate building blocks for dopamine, eat foods rich in Tyrosine. This amino acid can be found in almonds, bananas, avocados, eggs, beans, fish, and chicken.

Beyond a healthy diet and exercise, sleep is vital to getting your brain on track to heal itself. They all work in combination, rest, exercise and diet, to form the sustaining habits for the years ahead. The most important thing to remember is you can recover. No temporary setback of brain fogginess, fatigue or craving for stimulants need be permanent. Your future is wide open, once you leave behind the substances which are in your way.

–17–
HOW TO FIX THE OPIOID EPIDEMIC

As I write this, the world is fighting the Wuhan Corona virus. In the US, we've lost almost 200,000 souls, mostly in the setting of advanced age and multiple comorbidities. The virus from China preys on the elderly and infirm. Half of all deaths are patients who were in nursing homes (not the healthiest cohort). The average age of death is eighty; though some are under fifty. At the time of this writing, the virus appears to attack endothelial cells, abundant in the lungs. We have excellent treatments and a vaccine is on the horizon.

Opioid overdoses in the US were 67,000 last year (2019), an improvement from 71,000 the prior year. Over the past ten years, over 600,000 Americans died of opioid overdose. That's about as many as America lost in World War II. Unlike the SARS-CoV-2 virus, opioid overdose targets a much younger demographic. The 24-50-year-old group is most likely to die of an opioid OD. In terms of years of life lost, opioids are far more devastating than any Asian virus we've seen. We shut down the world for a pathogen that kills the sick and old, but we ignore the suicide and carnage wrought by opioids. It's time for change.

In Johann Hari's book *Chasing the Scream,* he describes the history of the war on drugs in the U.S. and worldwide. Hari outlines the history of prohibition in America. The "noble experiment" began in 1920. Though technically successful in reducing alcohol consumption, it was a very unpopular, leading to a wave of organized crime before it was repealed in 1933.

Harry Anslinger, head of the Office of Alcohol Control, found himself without a job. At the time, Indian Hemp (*Cannabis sativa*) was smoked sporadically by folks along our southwestern border. Though his stated positon on marijuana causing violence was, "There is probably no more absurd fallacy," he later backtracked and asked Congress for funding to go after marijuana dealers & customers. As it happened, they were mostly urban blacks.

Tireless in his police work against this cohort of Americans, he tracked down a small group, New York City jazz musicians who used heroin. He made an example of singer Nina Simone, and Hari's description of her death is heartbreaking. Masterful at fearmongering, Mr. Anslinger, portrayed heroin as the inevitable result of using marijuana. The concept of a gateway drug was born.

The ranks of Anslinger's deputies swelled, bristling with their mission: to stamp out marijuana and heroin in America. This was war. Heroin consumption was trivial overall; people were frightened of it. Marijuana use was uncommon: less than 5 percent of adults. Also, there was no significant organized crime activity yet around marijuana or opiates. Anslinger aggressively prosecuted anyone connected with drugs. Organized crime recognized the business opportunity after prohibition ended and shifted from selling alcohol to pushing drugs.

Anslinger was the leader of the war on drugs for 32 years, until he retired in 1963. He was a foreign ambassador of this policy too, forcing it on many other nations if they wanted to do business with the US. In many ways, we're still following the guidelines he laid down ninety years ago. Science and compassion have a long way to go if we want to undo Anslinger's legacy.

The premise of the war on drugs is intuitively simple and straightforward. It's not the person's responsibility for developing a substance habit, it's the drug which "hijacks" the victim's mind. Remember the Time Magazine cover from 1997 with a surreal fish/human chimera about to bite a sparkly hook? The artwork implies it's the drug turning a person into a mindless controlled zombie. In other words, if we could just get people to not use drugs, then addiction would never happen.

This is at odds with human nature, especially with how we manage discomfort. Nearly all animals use some sort of mind-altering substance to deal with life. Think of cats with catnip, or the drunk elephants. Certainly, as the most advanced creature on earth, we will modify our environment and seek the most intense high we can find. The mechanism of habit creation leaves it susceptible to the habit of using psychoactive substances. A tautological explanation: the drug causes the disease in the brain is plainly wrong. Only 10% of people who try *heroin* progress to a habit.

Tobacco (nicotine) is another example of why the "chemical hooks theory" is insufficient to explain the habit. It is common to hear quitting smoking is harder than quitting heroin. You know this isn't true. Prevalence of the smoking habit in the U.S. used to be two out of every three adults in 1960. This fell following the tobacco advertising ban and the surgeon general's warning in 1964. Change was slow, but change occurred.

Now the national average for tobacco dependence has gone from two out of three to less than one out of four, and it's headed down to one in of five. If tobacco really is more addictive than heroin, then how could you explain this national drop off of tobacco dependence rates?

Opioid medications like Vicodin, OxyContin, and morphine are prescribed for pain relief. In truth, their target is emotional more than physical. If you want to treat serious pain, anti-inflammatory drugs and local anesthetics (lidocaine) are much more effective. Opioids work differently– less on pain per se and more on the anguish of helplessness. Opioids reduce *suffering*. They help us tolerate a lack of choice, and they soften the sense of feeling trapped with our pain. No wonder we form habit loops in pursuit of this ease and comfort. Opioids make us feel better about our self-concept. Perhaps a few more words will help me explain.

We won't go too deep into theory of mind and the neural architecture of consciousness. But let's say how we imagine ourselves at least as critical as how we are in reality. We are not precisely what we think we are. Our understanding is less a hi-res photograph and more like a soft watercolor painting of the real world. Our minds, specifically the part of our mind that's aware of itself, is a bit like a motion picture screen showing a movie.

Professor Antonio Damasio, the distinguished neurologist from U.S.C. Medical School, writes in *Self Comes to Mind* about the internal brain-screen. He says upon it is "played" our sense experience and recalled memories. Each of us cobbles together a concept of individual identity in relation to the world about us. The human brain evolved from lower organisms, but the important ancient problems such as hunger, lust and fear are all still present and their systems are preserved.

For example, when hungry, you probably feel it in your stomach, or abdomen. But this is not where "hunger" is located. It is an ancient pathway triggered by *ghrelin*, the hunger hormone. Your brain makes up a story that your stomach is empty, and you're so used to the feeling, it's what hungry's come to mean. Opioid receptors decorate most of the organs of the body. Endogenous opioids (endorphins) calm and soothe pain. Feeling alright is what every organism craves; opioids are a shortcut to this feeling– a hack.

The opioid system was exploited by our ancestors. For millennia, our forebears ate and smoked extracts of *Papaver* whenever they could. Aristotle observed the poppy grows among the wheat; man's suffering is relieved alongside his hunger.

Since everyone wants to suffer less, it's easy to understand how opioids grew into an epidemic in the U.S. According to Nobel Laureate, Sir Angus Deaton, there is a socioeconomic drive which fuels the opioid epidemic. As the traditional framework of social order in modern society deteriorated, especially for white men, opioids were increasingly sought for relief of suffering. The economic damage caused by excessively Draconian lockdowns in response to the Wuhan Coronavirus is already causing a spike in suicide and a surge in drug use and overdoses.

Opioid use obviously doesn't make it easier to get a job, start a business, or be responsible enough to attract a mate and start a family. Opioids offer temporary respite from the self-loathing repeated failure engenders. We know they hurt us, but right now when we need it most, they take away the pain of uncertainty and doubt.

Drugs like opioids help you care less about your life falling apart, and this is why their use has boomed during the 21st century. Legal and economic pressure are worsened by a drug habit, and vice-versa. Geographically, the areas of steepest economic decline in the U.S. roughly correspond the wave of opioid-related deaths. Deaton and his co-researcher (and wife) Anne Case refer to this correlation as "deaths of despair." Suicide, drug overdose, and violence associated with drug use are all directly attributable to the life of the opioid addict in an economically depressed zone. Lack of meaning, loss of hope and suffering as all temporarily relieved with a dose of opioids.

Sam Quinones, the brilliant Los Angeles author of *Dreamland*, chronicles the rise of heroin use in America. Beginning in the Southwest, expanding into the Ohio and Kentucky, heroin overdoses tracked OxyContin prescriptions, especially from pill mills—shoddy medical practices with reputations for loose narcotic prescribing. Once patients were opioid habit hooked, according to Quinones, cheaper heroin allowed them to avoid painful withdrawal. It was supplied by industrious salesmen travelling up from Mexico in the form of black tar heroin.

It's incomplete to say prescription opiates themselves are the sole cause of the increase in heroin dependence. Prescription of opioids per capita peaked in 2006, but the overdose trend only started to slow its rise in 2018. Socioeconomic factors intensify pain avoidance; drug and alcohol use rises when an economy falls. Also note increased suicide disproportionately impacts men. Loss of identity, purpose, and social standing following loss of employment, not to mention disruption of family plans, are far more corrosive to one's self-image than a prescription for pain medicine. The opioid catastrophe took root in the fertile ground of globalization and off-shoring of American jobs. Another significant factor is our cultural attitude toward folks who develop a substance habit. Shunning them isn't helpful.

Muri Assunção writes in the May 6, 2019 edition of the NY Daily News:

In 1999, the small southern European country had the highest rate of drug-related AIDS in the European Union, the second highest prevalence of HIV among people who inject drugs, and an alarmingly increasing number of deaths by drug overdoses, according to a 2018 report by the U.S.-based organization Drug Policy Alliance.

A group of experts in substance addiction was assembled to come up with a plan to find a solution to the crisis. They proposed a bold and groundbreaking strategy, which included fully decriminalization. After it was approved by legislators in 2000, it went into effect in 2001.

The results are astounding: Heroin and cocaine use, two of the country's most worrying instances of substance abuse, went from 1% to 0.3%; HIV infections among drug users was reduced by 50%; In the general population HIV rate fell from 104 cases per million in 1999 to 4.2 in 2015. Drug-related incarceration also fell, from 75% to 45%, according to International Drug Policy Consortium (APDES), a non-profit that focus on drug policy and harm reduction.

Instead of continuing the disastrous war on drugs, let's declare an armistice. The war gave us the unintended opioid epidemic. Criminalizing habits and ruining the lives of those trapped by ignorance, economics and biology has failed. We tried prohibition but it only drove alcohol use into the speakeasies run by the mob.

The rise of the criminal underworld, gangs, and figures like Al Capone and Dutch Schultz, and later narco-traffickers like Pablo Escobar and Guzman are the natural result of fighting the human drive to relieve suffering. We can't let people free-feed opioids at the pharmacy with no restrictions; that won't work. So, what should we do?

The opioid epidemic in America is a *wicked problem*. This is not just Southie (Boston) slang, but a description of a type of problem that requires multiple stakeholders to cooperate, and with an end result that won't make anyone completely happy. From a law enforcement standpoint, officers and deputies want to get the criminals/bad guys, and prosecute all the drug dealers.

Average citizens want to keep drugs and alcohol out of the hands of children, and redirect interdiction resources toward better social services, but they also want to drink wine with dinner. Those with a drug habit want a solution for their suffering and sense of dispossession, they need meaning and purpose as well as discipline. Doctors want to treat disease, clergy want to offer guidance, drug kingpins want to live like Tony Montana. Some of these stakeholders and goals are at odds, clearly.

Hopelessness and despair correlate with the decline of the middle class in America. Economic improvement that reaches everyone would go a long way toward reducing the attraction of drugs and alcohol. Americans with an annual income of $20,000 or less (2011 figures), are three times more likely to have an opioid habit than is a countryman who earns over $40,000 per year. Improving the economy for the middle class is a far tougher challenge than locking up a few drug dealers.

Let's not forget the drug cartels either. They have developed an extensive business model in the U.S., as *Dreamland* describes, based roughly on the Domino's Pizza model of customer service. Under the cartel service model, you can get black tar heroin delivered to your door in thirty minutes or sooner. The distribution network is extensive and cellular; and large-volume/high-dollar drug busts are rare now.

Other advances from the business management, such as just-in-time inventory control, logistics, distributed processing, and empowering decision making at customer point of contact, have all had improved service by the drug cartels. In Mexico, the extent to which the multi-billion-dollar cartels have dominated political life is reflected in their private cellular communications network. The drug lords have cell towers carrying encrypted phone and text traffic on secure cartel devices. Electricians are forced at gunpoint to connect the shadow cell transmitters. Law enforcement doesn't mess with the communications network. They are either paid to ignore the cartels, or simply want to avoid being shot. *Plata* or *plomo* in Spanish–in English: silver or lead. If we ignore cartel stakeholders (and their government backers), we won't be able to solve our wicked problem. Cartels will exploit any opportunity and service their customer base, unless our solution addresses the conditions which allow cartels to thrive we'll continue to be doomed.

You can see simply interdicting the drug itself hasn't won't ever work. Desperation finds a workaround. Not one more child should become dependent on drugs. Unfortunately, liberalizing access means more kids will develop a substance problem. If drugs are easier to get, more people will try them. Look at the marijuana use data following legalization if you still aren't convinced.

Once you accept these premises, the question becomes, "If people have an addiction habit, how do we help them?" Presently, they are still shamed and ostracized from society. Help is limited usually to prison, expensive medical treatment, or further misguided efforts at deterrence. Even after stopping a drug or alcohol habit, stigma remains. Prospective employers upon learning of prior substance use, are reluctant to hire even the recovered substance user.

One estimate of gross *profit* from the opioid epidemic flows into Mexico at a rate of over $50 billion per year. Our cartel stakeholders won't surrender this river of gold without a fight. Imagine the cost in terms of human suffering this industry imposes on the innocent as well as the guilty.

Although it makes many Americans uneasy to contemplate, we should consider the success of the Portuguese experiment in decriminalization. Instead of fighting reality, let us recognize it is normal to seek relief from pain–emotional as well as physical. Critics of the experiment in Portugal point to the increase in people who've ever tried drugs. This is an unavoidable consequence or removing criminal penalties for drug use. But the rate of overdose, the proportion of the incarcerated who have drug problems, HIV prevalence, and medical costs for the habituated population have all fallen dramatically.

Opioid dependence is not a foe that can be forced into submission. You're dealing with millions of years of evolution which have crafted our habit-loop systems. We're not going to outsmart the brain, but knowing how it works you can outsmart your addiction. The best we can hope for is a truce, a negotiated peace. We must recognize some people are bent toward habits with self-destructive ends; others are not.

If we direct all of our resources trying to fight addiction, we will fail. If we prosecute the person who has developed a drug or alcohol habit, we'll be right back to square one. To win the war over alcohol and drugs, we must realize habits account for our success as a species. We must treat each other with tender compassion and loving accountability if we really want to succeed.

A big reason for lower crime in Portugal: it's now safe for the habituated to get help. They know they won't be arrested, or lose their jobs, so they come in. They come in for drug testing, HIV testing and treatment, medical care, and even mobile testing at large gatherings so people can find out what their street drugs are really cut with.

This is another reason to decriminalize drug use and make the drugs available in a clinical setting. Thousands die every year from accidental overdose. With the phenomenon of tolerance, over time they develop a stable opioid use pattern. If the habituated can't find their usual supply, they grab what they can. The black market for substances has no federal purity or labeling standards.

It's east to take for granted the pharmacy fills the prescription ordered by your doctor. People who get their drugs from the street aren't so confident. Heroin, is cut (diluted with inert ingredients like sugar), often several times. Occasionally, dealers will spike a batch and use that as a marketing tool, as we've discussed earlier. Current habitual customers ask the dealer for "the same stuff she had." The intention is not to overdose, but mistakes happen in manufacturing all the time.

If instead, as is done in England, Switzerland and Portugal, users could receive opioids as a public benefit of the state, they would know for sure what drugs they're using. Overdose risk plummets, and if people are treated decently they tend to participate willingly.

I know talking about legalization or decriminalization is going to be met with resistance in the US. In considering all stakeholders, law enforcement is among the largest and most important. Forgoing asset confiscation policies will cost local enforcement millions. Also, the "prison industrial complex," if there is such an entity, is most profitable at high marginal occupancy. Drug addicts are the best prisoners: easily managed, relatively docile in captivity, and controllable with a contraband market of substances. As a result, prison personnel costs and employee retention improve with fewer sociopathic criminals in the general population. Legal and corrective institutions also resist change.

A pilot program would be ideal, and best in a specific hard-hit area. Training programs, work opportunities, and improvement in the local economy would combine to help the local population develop purpose, mission, and to change substance habits. Though there will be an increase in first-time users, we should nevertheless decriminalize consumption for personal use.

You can expect pushback from the drug dealers, their business model disrupted, but also from the legal system invested in the war on drugs. Once successful in a several tests, let's try it in a state like Rhode Island or New Hampshire, where opiate deaths per capita are among the highest in the country. If these programs continue to be successful, then we might roll out *anti-prohibition* for the whole country.

And finally, the best thing we can do is to stop altogether calling addiction a *disease*. I hope the pages of this book, the references to our animal kin in the wild, the stories of redemption, have coalesced to help you see this problem with new eyes. It's anything but a disease in my opinion. A habit, yes. One that can feel automatic, surely, especially in the context of tolerance and withdrawal. But calling it a disease doesn't help you to get off your duff and change the things you can. Speaking of which, let's look a little bit more closely at spirituality in the next chapter. There is something we can surely change.

–18–

SPIRITUALITY AND ADDICTION

Matters of the spirit are always intensely personal. And as nurturing as spirituality can be, disagreements about it are also the basis of countless conflicts. Potter Stewart's remark about things everyone knows but which are hard to define, "I know it when I see it," applies in full measure to matters of the spirit. Religion is the ritual and ordered practice of underlying spirituality. Most of us carry at least a few religious notions, even if we don't attend regular services. Even those who declaim a higher power, most always have an appreciation for the unseen, be it nature, mathematics, or simply the mysterious.

A simple definition for religion/God/higher power is *what you value highest*. At one point, I valued alcohol and drugs most highly. Is this your experience too? My days were organized around the ritual of acquiring, experiencing, and recovering from my habitual use of chemicals. The most devout acolyte had nothing on my fervor to use a chemical coping strategy.

If we regard something with topmost value, we supinate before its influence on our behavior. For example, if the most important thing to you is exercise, then you will probably be "religious" about it. Your day will be arranged around making sure you get to the gym. If exercise is not your highest aspiration or driving force, if it is not your "religion," you'll likely skip the workout. I used to jettison exercise like disposable ballast during stressful times; I know better now.

The same idea can apply to almost anything you focus on habitually. Food, sex, work, collecting stamps, collecting cars, or any repetitive activity you can think of. You need only look at the diversity of religious practices to see we can make meditation, physical labor, chanting, or building a mandala out of sand in order to channel the power of our attention.

All religions exploit the human yearning for an explanatory model of the world, a way to make sense of the mysterious. Imponderables like: why are we here? what is the meaning of life? and what happens when we die? are all profound questions that so far remain unanswered by man. One of my professors— the man who gave me a second chance in anesthesiology, Dr. Peter Moore—had a mental filing system for problems like these. He'd put them in a "box" in his mind labeled "too hard." The kind of problems that won't yield to thinking; we were never going to come up with a satisfactory answer. We try anyway, but get no closer to untangling the knots. Too hard.

Spirituality is inseparable from the history of substance habit treatment, and runs through virtually every modern rehab system. The "12-step model" is dominant, serving as the core 93 percent of treatment centers in the U.S. Even those that do not use the 12-step model, such as Narcanon (Scientology), all employ a religious framework in which to understand addiction.

For the skeptical, appeals to spirituality or a higher power sound a lot like "trust us." This feels inconceivable to someone new to the concept of habit change. Habitual substance users have been wronged by caregivers or family mistrust the Universe. For them the world of people is full of dirty tricks. When advised trust in a fellow human being is the path to saving themselves, they flinch from the suggestion. Submitting oneself to a set of laws (including spiritual axioms), as Cicero described, is essential. We must function in an ordered society with boundaries and expectations of conduct. Religious ideas or spiritual principles are the synthetic residue of lives well lived—or poorly lived—throughout human history.

To break the "spell" of drugs and alcohol you must confide in at least one other person. "Trust the process," is a tough pill to swallow. Who hasn't been burned, wronged, or betrayed by those closest? I've heard it said our mental representation of God is anchored by our experience of our parents. If they failed us at critical moments during our upbringing, it leaves a residue of mistrust. Verbal and physical abuse, neglect, and parental self-absorption with substance habits all leave deep emotional scars that persist into adulthood. If you were raised by substance-dependent parent it can feel as if you were raised by a crazy person. If you *are* a substance dependent parent, it's time to change.

When a child grows up in a chaotic environment, she launches into the adult world wracked with self-doubt. Poor self-esteem is the result, unfortunately often manifested in deprecation of others. Alcoholics Anonymous recommends newcomers connect with more experienced members. They have a special term for the person who shows the newbie around a sober life: sponsor.

Sponsors don't provide financial help; they provide guidance and nonjudgmental support. With consistency, luck, and some small part of skill on the part of the sponsor, a relationship is fostered. If you can find one person with whom you can safely be honest, you have more than a fighting chance to break a substance habit.

This reminds me of the scene in *The Little Prince* between the prince and the fox. Antoine de Saint-Exupéry's classic decocts the perfect parable of trust between the timorous mammal and the curious boy. Humans are predators to foxes. Yet, longing for contact, each seeks to bridge the gulf of fear and distrust.

The fox, eager to be tamed, tells the little prince how to go about it. He advises that they meet at the same time, each day at four o'clock. The fox explains, initially it'll be on guard, and won't even dare approach the boy. But if the boy is consistent and patient and keeps showing up the same time every day, eventually the fox will come to expect his arrival.

As the fox grows more accustomed to the pattern of the boy's regular appointment, it will venture a little bit closer every time to the rock where the boy sits. The fox continues, knowing that the boy is coming at four, it will begin to get excited around 3:45. Then, with more consistency, the fox will get excited at half past three, and so on. This is how they become the best of friends. Though literary fantasy, the method of establishing trust, and redemption, works in recovery when you need to make real contact.

Consistency is key.

Alcoholics Anonymous adopted a prayer attributed to Reinhold Niebuhr, but it probably was uttered long before he did. The *Serenity Prayer*: "God, grant me serenity to accept the things I cannot change, courage to change the things I can, and the wisdom to know the difference."

This tripartite prayer is the greatest filing system of all time (Thanks Frank B). Let's break down the components. There are things *outside* of our control; that's most of the Universe. These include the seasons, the tide, the weather, and (crucially) every person, place or thing that isn't you. Certainly, the past is outside of anyone's control, but *what we think about the past* is in the next category.

Fortunately, the important stuff is *within* our command. Our attitudes and actions may seem insignificant compared with all that's beyond our reach. But few ever come close to efficient use of the time and ability they possess. We squander so much of what we've been given. If we could only focus all of our efforts on actions in our ambit, and stop trying to control what we can't, there's no telling what each of us could do. Sorting which action goes in which bin—that's the third part of the prayer: the *wisdom to know the difference.*

Unfortunately, we all have blind spots, part of the purpose of religion or a spiritual practice is to help us see our blind spots. Better, to respond to them in real-time with more efficient effort than we might come up with on our own. We consult the ancient texts and stories which point the way. Heroes who behaved appropriately despite fear, and villains who took shortcuts each have something to teach.

If you flip the Serenity Prayer and instead seek courage to change the things we <u>can't</u> and the serenity sit back when <u>action is imperative</u>, you have the recipe for misery. America is suffering from an obesity pandemic. On a demographic scale, we consume more calories than we work off. America is not alone, obesity's plaguing most wealthy countries. We eat our feelings, we eat as habit, and this practice is made all the more appealing by wizard chefs in our food and beverage industries. Despite all, we remain ultimately responsible for the reading on the bathroom scale.

No person is *required* to eat more than she or he should. We let things slide today because an extra slice of pizza doesn't seem to make much difference. Add an extra 500 calories a day for a year though, and you'll gain more than *thirty* pounds.

Similarly, <u>one day at a time</u> is a powerful idea and a slogan from AA. This nugget of philosophy takes things in small enough bites so we aren't overwhelmed by worry concerning the future. Thinking about things in small segments—just one day—allows us to forgive our prior mistakes and look at things with fresh eyes. To turn the page.

Wisdom to know the difference is augmented by perspective and wise counsel from our close friends/family. Ever had spinach in your teeth but you didn't know? It's embarrassing to be told our smile is festooned with greens, but worse to find out later in the mirror, after your big date.

If you cultivate a few friends you can trust, and you are candid with them, you'll make fewer mistakes. Opening up and being honest with a few good men is one of the best early-sobriety decisions I made. Gentlemen, thanks for your wisdom, guidance and love.

Choose well your inner circle; people can take unfair advantage of you in these situations. To receive genuine help, you have to be genuine yourself. But your candor doesn't guarantee the person you open up to will be of high ethical caliber. Anyone who'd use your honesty to harm you must be avoided. Though bottled up secrets will fester, you still have to choose carefully the company you keep.

Simply knowing that you *have* blind spots is helpful. In my car, the right side-view mirror has a warning at the bottom: Objects may be closer than they appear. We must consider the context for the ideas we hold, especially about ourselves. Even though a car may look small, and far away, the wide field of view afforded by the convex shape of the mirror has to be taken into account. Our own distorted perceptions confer an advantage under certain circumstances, but can cause us to miscalculate risk and reward.

Another favorite concept from the world of addiction recovery is GOD—an acronym for Good Orderly Direction. I'll stay out of theology in this chapter, but *direction* is simply knowing what we need to do to get where we want to go. We need to know which way to go or we'll never get anywhere. Sometimes, what I thought was a great idea sounds more like a flop once I share it (honestly) with others. They point out the holes in my thinking, the blind spots, and often will share their experience with a similar problem. I've made a lot of mistakes in my personal life, but far fewer once I asked my personal board of directors.

Remember the Rat Park story? The little varmints in tiny cages rapidly developed a habit loop for drug/alcohol/electric zaps. Reintroduced to a more normal rat society, they abandoned their addictions. In a funny way, I'm encouraging you to make your own Rat Park. Amass a collection of good people who support your success. If you're lucky, you'll share a common experience trying to do the best you can with the limits of this thing called life. Associating with people like this–people on a mission of personal development–is in an experience not to be missed. Stick with the winners.

I'm an evangelical for *practical spirituality*. I imagine the Universe is a loving place, but it is also harsh if I fail to follow The Rules. If I do my best, tell the truth, lend a hand, ask for help, and be part of the solution, this puts me in an open and receptive frame of mind. I become more present, and I'm able to participate in the unfolding events at hand without running to a chemical.

If instead I think that the universe is random, stochastic, and uncaring place, I'll imagine the world from a scared, defensive point of view. Alienation from my fellows, as Nietzsche described, is the road to personal corruption and a disintegration of society. Nietzsche in the 19th Century, predicted the horrors of the 20th if society continued to reject the deeper order of the world. Startlingly, he foresaw the rise of Nazi Germany, Soviet Russia, and the Great Leap Forward in China. Combined, these three "advances" of socialism/communism are responsible for the deaths of 100,000,000 souls. When we lose our sense of community and right conduct, the Universe will soon bring us to ruin.

Don't worry, you can be an atheist/agnostic and still change your habits to suit yourself. Even as a man of science, I found we each must believe in *something*, even if it is gravity waves, dark matter, or an infinitely iterated fractal. Nobody believes in *nothing*. We each have some inner belief, otherwise our suffering would be meaningless.

We transmute our experience from the base to the precious when we speak honestly to those we value. We redeem ourselves every time we tell the truth. A line from the "promises" section of the AA book says we will *not regret the past, nor wish to shut the door on it*. We come to see our behaviors from a new vantage. When we do, helped by our community, we are redeemed.

–19–
MY OWN SPIRITUAL AWAKENING

Inpatient residential treatment is a luxury most people cannot afford. Besides the cost, few can comfortably take a month (or more) away from their responsibilities. Perhaps, some day, it will be replaced with a brief period of medical and social stabilization, followed by long-term support. This would mimic the overwhelmingly successful diversion programs. In the future, readers of this book may wonder why anyone ever went "away" for help to change a habit. Prior to working in the field for nearly two decades, I also went to rehab. In the next story, I'll share with you the best of what can happen inside of a residential treatment facility (rehab).

I was a guest of Springbrook Northwest in Newberg, Oregon, for three months commencing in January in 2000. Today this rehab is part of the Hazelden-Betty Ford system. Atypically, I was abstinent from drugs and alcohol for three months before checking in. My adventure in unmedicated home detox is chronicled earlier in this book. Despite demonstrating I could get and stay sober, the California Diversion program mandated a stint in a sanctioned facility. I showed up to check that box.

Ninety days was the minimum standard commitment in rehab for a physician. Likely, the custom was more about revenue (physicians can typically afford the fees) than about public safety. Longer stays in rehab *per se* do not equal higher chance of abstinence. I've never seen those data. There is a correlation between longer <u>total time</u> in a structured program, but the fraction of that time in a residential rehab is at best irrelevant. It may even be detrimental. Despite the logically inconsistent rule, there was no way for me to stay for fewer days: who was I to argue?

Since I couldn't truncate my stay, I decided to get the most I could out of it. I understood drugs and alcohol were in my past. Given the damage they caused me, there was no way to rationalize the risk of picking them up again. I had a hard time dealing with my feelings of inadequacy. I also was mixed up and had an unclear life direction. Maybe the counselors and the system would help me find the way forward. I was open to the process, but intensely skeptical any of this would work.

Concepts like spirituality, higher power, and honesty were foreign to me. I also had a contrarian streak which manifested in intense dislike for order and rules. The 12 steps themselves appeared an embodiment of a fascist police state; commandments imposed on me by caprice from a far-off New York office. You get the picture: I was a defiant young doctor. Maybe my intravenous narcotic use has already conveyed this trait.

At Springbrook, we patients filled out worksheets and shared our stories in the manner inspired by the twelve steps of A.A. In 1934, Bill Wilson, the stockbroker who co-founded A.A., during his final detox for alcohol withdrawal, experienced hallucinations enhanced by belladonna prescribed by his psychiatrist. Wilson, at the time, was a member of the Oxford group: a religious temperance organization with a six-step sobriety plan.

He attempted to get sober via Oxford, but found himself again hospitalized and near death. During the DTs/drug hallucinations, the salesman experienced a revelation. Wilson improved on Oxford by doubling the number of steps to twelve. If he only knew his musings would became the of commandments every treatment center group room.

I went along for the rehab ride, playing the role of enthusiastic participant. Candidly though, I was cynical about any brief indoctrination having a lasting effect. I'd already kicked dope, and I paid lip-service when the counselors prodded me to say I wouldn't drink alcohol. I'd been careful to never let booze get out of hand. I had zero expectations that rehab would fix anything important. I knew myself well, and made it this far without surrendering my core self-concept: irreparably damaged. Your skeptical doctor signed up for treatment as a practical matter, so I could keep my medical license.

Our assignments logically began with Step One, *we admitted we were powerless over alcohol – that our lives had become unmanageable.* Put another way, it means we're helpless to control our intake of substances and alcohol once we start drinking/using. We each wrote and shared about our experiences, especially those when we planned to have a couple of drinks but wound up drunk. The point of the exercise is to highlight the mechanism of neural control by ethanol. Once the drug is taken, the mind changes plans. From "let's have one," to "let's close down the bar." This is straightforward and wasn't particularly threatening. The words after the dash are a bit tougher.

Unmanageability, I assumed, is a natural consequence of chronic substance use. A messy, dissipated life, and the inability to handle day-to-day tasks, flows from wasting so much time on getting wasted. Eventually I'd understand unmanageability as referenced has nothing to do with dependence on substances. Actually, it's the failure to live by a set of personal rules, corner-cutting, that damages relationships and makes simple tasks feel overwhelming; unmanageable. But at that point, at least I could clearly comprehend that life was better without fentanyl. Thus, step one handled, I bade farewell to opioids and other drugs.

Step two: *We came to believe that a power greater than ourselves could restore us to sanity.* Woah. This is another way of saying YOU'RE NUTS! Not just nuts, but a special kind of nuts that only a supernatural being can fix. This was a much harder pill to choke down. First, the higher power idea to me at the time was reserved for the weak-minded. They proposed I should believe in mystical white-bearded geezer up in heaven; sure, that's what the counselors were saying. Stubbornly, I held firm. The second part of Step Two, "restore us to sanity," was double stupid. What insane person graduates from Berkeley, medical school, surgical internship, and completes two-thirds of an anesthesia residency? You can't be nuts and do all of that, right?

This step called for a deeper think. Okay, shooting fentanyl is hard to categorize as rational behavior, that I could concede. Besides the constant risk of infection, death itself comes easily on the wings of an overdose. On a long enough timeline, everyone's survival falls to zero, but shooting dope foreshortens it. I never contemplated suicide. I was using drugs for relief of emotional pain and got caught up in a habit cycle. Unfortunate, perhaps, but not crazy. Still, with a clear mind it was hard to explain my choice of remedy for emotional self-rejection. I scoffed; how could I be *insane?*

But in more open, reflective moments, I could see there was no other way to describe my self-destructive and pointless risk-taking. Instead of doing something simple (and sane) like asking for help, or saying aloud "I'm scared," I forged ahead and told no one. "Knowing better," I still shot chemicals into my veins. A dangerous notion still lurked in my mind: *once Diversion is over I'll go back to drinking–recreationally.* I harbored this idea, conceding injectable opiates were out but no one could deny me a glass of scotch after a hard day at the office.

I created a psychological stash, a backdoor to relief. I kept my secret belief in a liquid chemical higher power. I counted on it to get me through the tough times of the future. Since rehab was an empty compliance exercise, when it was over at least I could drink like a gentleman.

I examined more closely this irrational, entitled idea. Mercifully, I caught the break of a lifetime. In what I'm sure was an epiphany, I understood this *drink-someday* idea was potentially lethal. What else but crazy to conclude that just because I had some pleasant prior experiences with alcohol, I could switch chemicals to escape reality? How could I live *without alcohol* but also require it to *survive?*

There is a word to describe my mental pretzel-logic: insanity. Talk about whiplash to my tender self-image! Thus, the honest answer: all chemicals had to go. I'd simply been *wrong* about requiring something (a drug) to survive. And with that erroneous loop cut, my whole Christmas sweater of crazy came unraveled. With a flash of insight, I never had to repeat the experiment of using chemical to manage my feelings again. I was free.

If I could be wrong about something I was so sure of (alcohol is necessary for my survival) what else could I be mixed up about? I was mistaken about rehab having nothing to offer. Here it was working in real-time in my life. Could I be wrong about *thinking there was something wrong with me?* I had jumped to a mistaken conclusion as a child, and refused to let go of my "certain" knowledge. It was also evident I'd needed help to discover my error; the rehab, diversion, Dr. Moore and Fentanyl all helped me see where I was in error. Me plus others, <u>a power greater than myself</u>, had restored me to sanity.

It was winter in Oregon. Inside the stuffy rehab bungalow, working on my Step Two worksheet, I was overcome with emotion. Feeling hot, I went outside for some fresh air. A few steps outside the building I knelt in the damp cold grass under an old plane tree, boughs festooned with crows. I felt stupid and smart at the same time. Smart for letting go of an old idea, stupid for clutching it so long. I could see clearly my own foibles, silly self-reliance on my own judgment. In fear, I clung to a self-destructive lie. It was time to let it go and I promised myself I'd face reality without chemicals. I began to cry *and laugh* at the same time.

Huge shuddering sobs mixed with convulsions laughter; it was the most intense emotional and spiritual experience I'd had. As I chucked and sobbed, the inky avian chorus joined in chiding me. There on my knees under a leafless tree, the Universe thoughtfully arranged for a murder of crows help me kill my hubris. In that moment, understanding flooded in: I am just a person. I get things wrong. I make mistakes. I'm not a mistake.

The case I make here is for a practical spirituality. Since we can't know, why not give the idea that there's more to life than we can see a try? Meaning is created when by our focus of attention. When I think about a higher order, an organizing force, I feel better and am more useful to others. If I stay out of the debate about the existence of a higher power, I'm free to experience one. Give it a try, you might be surprised how helpful this practical attitude is. Free of my pernicious limiting belief, I reexamined my entire personal philosophy.

Perhaps I'd been wrong about my father. I came to understand he was also a man with his own challenges and fears. He used alcohol and relationships to attempt to reconcile his sense of inadequacy. Now that I understood we are all inadequate as individuals, there wasn't anything defective about me which needed fixing. Same for my father; he wasn't able to accept himself as a work in progress. He rejected himself as unworthy and that stance colored all of his relationships the same way it had affected all of mine. I forgave him because I was able to forgive myself.

If my father and I were just two human beings doing the best we could with limited information, that concept was easily extended to my mother. She had enormous challenges growing up, health issues, and she fell in love with a troubled man. If we were all trying to get by, then she was as well.

Instead of judging he to a standard of perfection which I'd rejected myself for failing to achieve, I opened my heart and forgave her too.

And it turns out, forgiveness is a gift, but it is a gift you give yourself. Dropping my disapproval and resentment, laughing with the mocking crows, I was able to appreciate the sacrifices made by others on my behalf. My courage led to the epiphany and with the new knowledge my whole world changed. I had an entirely new way of seeing the world. I'd developed a new philosophy.

–20–
CULTIVATING YOUR PERSONAL PHILOSOPHY

Spending thoughtful effort to craft your personal philosophy is critical. Whether you deliberately crafted it or not, you have one. If you're like I was, your default assumptions about yourself and your place in the world don't get much of your conscious attention. I drifted for years living what Socrates called the unexamined life. Each of us surely approaches the world in a specific way and we have our individual own code of personal conduct. The most important element is what you think about the world and about yourself in it. Your philosophy is the foundation stone of your happiness or sadness.

Most think philosophy is the dry writing of ancients such as Socrates or Plato. Fuzzy-headed and indecipherable, the word philosophy alone has frightened off many from its fruits. Let's end the myth that only sophisticated academics can assemble a personal philosophy. Every one of us has a philosophy, a general set of guidelines and principles, which cover what we think of ourselves and our relationships to others. An example may help.

We have a small family pet, a Bichon-Frise dog, named Lola, and two King Charles Spaniels, Rex & Belle. Family and dogs together all live near a scrubland California State Park area which is home to countless packs of coyotes. Our dogs bark at the window whenever a coyote passes through the backyard. Their gruff display is all warning bluster, and the wild and the domestic canines are separated by a backyard fence.

Coyotes are always hungry and on the prowl for a meal. One day our pets were barking at the back window, requesting to go outside in the yard. They thus signaled their need to "do their chore," but on this day, something else troubles the pooches. Lola ran outside to her patch of grass, and was screaming and barking across the back fence as loudly as she could. Moments later a large coyote vaulted the fence and grabbed Lola's head between its grizzled teeth. The maw of the wild beast was so big that the whole head of our little Lola disappeared inside.

Each of our three dogs has its own human. The two spaniels "belong" to my wife and me, and the Bichon is bonded more to our son. I was at work during coyotegate, and it was my wife who leapt to action to save Lola. The coyote, over one hundred pounds and standing three and a half feet at crown of its skull, had Lola in its mouth as it prepared to leap back over the fence to its—though not Lola's—safety.

Mrs. Giles grabbed the small dog around Lola's shoulders with one hand, and with her other, balled up a tight fist and wailed on the coyote's snout. The coyote was stunned, and stood there taking repeated blows. My wife suffered many nicks and cuts in her hand from the sharp teeth and barbed whiskers of the intruder. Calculating the meal too costly, the coyote opened its mouth, surrendering the prize. The savior gave the coyote a few more going-away smacks, and it clambered back over the fence. Lola sustained only a small tear underneath the chin. No stitches, no infection, and the rabies vaccinations were up to date.

My wife's philosophy is evident in this tale: protect the critters you care about, even at personal risk. She didn't ponder for second whether the coyote would attack her. It was going to eat Lola without her muscular intervention. She gave it her all, not just for the protection of our small animal, but so our son would not lose his beloved dog.

Lola had her own epiphany and philosophic reframing that morning. She previously had been aggressive in the yard, yelling at anything that she didn't like. After this experience, she became far more cautious. It's difficult to get her to even go outside now. Her philosophy adapted interaction with something large and scary outside of her normal routine. Today she is wary, and stays close when outdoors.

The Skinnerites (Followers of Dr. BF Skinner who believe environment determines behavior) would say Lola's change is nothing more than behavioral adaptation to a stimulus. I differ with their viewpoint. Lola, before encountering the coyote, had some idea about what interacting with a large beast would be like. She thought if she simply barked enough, a coyote would slink away. Imagine the shock when she found herself halfway down the beast's throat. Also, while my wife would've said beforehand that she would defend Lola against the coyote, I think she surprised herself with her mama-bear toughness toward the trespasser. My wife found another chunk of her inner badass.

A personal philosophy, influences all decisions. You're usually not aware of its pull, but it can be revealed at certain moments. Philosophy drives action at the deepest subconscious levels. These internal rules can be modified, and under drastic circumstances, completely revised. You can think of it as a motto if you like. For the longest time, my core personal philosophy was *I'm not good enough.*

I thought there was something about me which was either faulty, busted, or just missing. This is a hell of a way to live. Lack of self-worth led to self-loathing which led to medicine for my pain. I compounded my error with a second one: if I could only *learn enough,* I could overcome the defect I was born with. My inadequacy was fuel to vanquish academic challenges. A practical benefit of my insanity, I suppose. I certainly had a lot of external praise for my academic accomplishments, but this approbation never seemed to penetrate my calloused self-disregard.

Also, the sense that I wasn't good enough drove my drug use. Feeling less-than, is emotionally painful. Substances became a matter of survival, and a physical confirmation of my philosophy. The Imposter Syndrome roughly describes the deep sense on unworthiness I felt. Ancient texts talk of original sin: a mark that can't be washed off.

Many psychologists focus on childhood trauma and attachment theory, which says separation is the cause of the deepest wound. They're both useful models, but I believe perception of trauma is more important than the trauma per se. In other words, what we think and how we feel about the past drives us more than the actual events themselves. Belief might as well be reality. If you believe had a crummy childhood, then *you did,* whether or not a neutral observer would agree with your account.

I'll go out on a limb a little to suggest, you probably know someone who suffered as a child. I hope the person you're thinking of could find some aspects of his or her life for which they are grateful. The enemy of gratitude is blame. I spent years trying to assign responsibility for my shortcomings to someone else; some of my outlook was rooted in my rough upbringing. I practiced feeling like a victim, and I laid the blame on my parents. These were the attitudes and the emotional maturation of a child. It's human nature to make a list of excuses why we failed when we don't get something we want. I wanted a good life, to feel secure and confident, and above all like I belonged. Couldn't be **I** had anything to do with how my life went, right?

People are exceptionally creative at placing the responsibility on anyone but themselves for their situation. We blame the government, taxes, Republicans, Democrats, our parents, the economy, etc. Anything that is slightly plausible will work its way into a defense narrative for why we're not where we should be. A popular comment in politics is to say the other guy is "dividing the people." The implication being we should all come together, but under MY rule. A difference of political opinion is transformed into "sewing division." Fortunately, most people see through that ploy. Calls for "unity" nowadays mean "you are wrong, join my side."

Speaking of politics, maybe you heard there was an upset in a recent national election in America. One candidate, certain she was going to win, lost. Afterward, she published a book accounting for her failure. It amounted to nothing more than a book-length list of blame and excuses. Success has a thousand parents, but failure is an orphan. Blaming is human nature and, ironically, may be one of the few humanizing aspects of her *apologia.*

Who can't relate to feeling less-than and blaming other people for our own shortcomings? But when examined carefully, where does our habit of blame get us? If you believe that you are the primary actor in your life, the agent that gets things done, then blaming others takes you out of position of power. Late comedian Jonathan Winters said, "If your ship doesn't come in, *swim out to meet it.*"

People who are passive and wait for others to take care of them, do for them, and make everything okay, are inevitably miserable. We are built to reach, strive, and try to be better. Take writing this book, for example. I've known I needed to get these ideas out for a long time. For many years I have been working on this, mulling the idea of telling the truth about myself and how I see this addiction problem differently from a disease. It's intimidating to take on the dominant view of anything, addiction included.

Resistance, the inner voice distracting and blocking you from accomplishing anything great. Beautifully described by Steven Pressfield, in *The War of Art*, my own resistance was hard to deal with every time I sat down to write this book. Pushing through, disciplining myself to write even though I worried about getting my ideas out into the big wide world, was hard but worth it.

Unless I told my inner critic to shut up, you wouldn't be reading these words. Human beings are less afraid of being *meaningless* than they are of being *meaningful*. Dorothea Brand, in her book *Wake Up and Live*, accurately describes the will-to-failure. It goes hand-in-glove with the will to *blame*. We make our own meaning out of the material of our experiences. What we tell ourselves and our personal conduct are enormously important.

If our lives are meaningless, if we are just microscopic bits of stardust floating in the void, then it doesn't really matter what we do. Our failures and successes are irrelevant, and a personal philosophy I hear a lot is, "it is what it is." Another one I hear frequently: "What difference will it make in a thousand years?" These are nihilistic philosophies taken to the extreme. If we have no traction or tangible work product in our lives, then what we do truly is irrelevant. If this is the case, then drinking or trashing your life with drugs is quite a reasonable option, because at least doing so briefly distracts you while you're hurtling toward the black hole of nothingness.

No, people are terrified of their lives *having meaning*. This implies everything they do is judged. The sleight of hand trick of blaming your failures on someone else is spotted every time. The important issue is what you think about yourself. If you have tried to do something, if you have given it your whole heart and honest effort, then you will be transformed by the process. It matters not whether you reach your goal, but that in your effort you learn what you're made of. It's the *attempt* at making meaning that makes the meaning.

We *all* experience trauma at some point. Everyone has events and disappointments that they wish didn't happen. Many believe that their childhood has permanently damaged their adulthood. That their yesterdays have ruined all their tomorrows. That someone else, not you, controls and defines how your adult life works out. This is a lie and you should abandon it now if you've been telling yourself this falsehood. We all have circumstances and challenges, but you have controlling input into the direction of your life. The right plan (direction) plus time will take you anywhere you want to go. It's not too late to have a happy childhood.

Some use daily affirmations as prayers, concrete reminders of the direction they want to trudge, of the philosophy they wish to embrace. People write down where they want to be, or what their goals are. Frequent affirmations are, "I am rich," or "I am skinny."

This is all fine to have a goal, and to remind ourselves where we're headed. But just as important might be to write down, "I am fat," or "I am broke." Maybe make a little card that says Ï have a chemical habit to manage my feelings." Stick that on the bathroom mirror or put it on the dashboard of your car. Confront yourself with a splash of reality.

Rookie slugging sensation Aaron Judge was a September call-up in 2016. He was signed by the New York Yankees because he has tremendous bat speed and blasts monster home runs. He is a power hitter and plays decent right field too.

Aaron Judge's first month of plate appearances in the big leagues was far short of Yankee expectations. He had flashes of brilliance, but finished the season with a dismal batting average of 0.189.

He wrote down this number, 0.189, and carried it with him throughout the whole off season. This is like the baseball equivalent of writing down, "I am fat." Instead of saying, "I'm a great Yankee slugger and I can hit the ball really far." Writing down the truth of a sub-200 batting average was a tangible reminder he was below expectations for a big-leaguer.

If Judge failed to improve he'd be released. He wrote the truth rather than a fantasy aspiration. Consequently, he worked harder. The truth did set him free: free to mash. Judge came back in the spring of 2017 and went on to break the rookie home run record in his first full season. He knew where he was, *and* where he wanted to be.

Where are you hitting 0.189 in your life? How's your relationship with your spouse? How are things going with your coworkers? Are you honest with your friends? Do people know where you stand and are you someone who is reliable in a jam? When I asked myself these questions, I didn't like the answers. For a long time, I covered up my accurate sense of shortcoming with alcohol and drugs. This solution, I don't need to remind you, fails every time.

In order to cultivate your own philosophy, you must begin by being honest with yourself. No more self-deception, no more chemicals to muddy your accurate self-assessment. Once you have a clear picture, you can reflect on your choices, their results, and where you want to be in the future.

Then go back and, if you like, read what Socrates had to say. Here's one of my favorites:

"Smart people learn from everything and everyone, average people from their experiences, stupid people already have all the answers."

−21−
THE WAY FORWARD

Ever stayed up all night worrying about something coming with the dawn? There is an old Laurel & Hardy scene with the comedy duo in captured in wartime and stuck in prison. Stan, too anxious to mentally process the camp commandant's execution orders—the pair are to be shot at dawn—he asks his buddy, Oliver "what did he say?" The big guy repeats the grim sentence, and Laurel tearfully remarks, "I hope it's cloudy tomorrow."

Sometimes dread can be so severe the mind can find no peaceful place to light. I was terrified the night before my first day of internship at the hospital. Though excited to finally be a "real doctor" on the hospital wards, I feared screwing up.

In the better part of two decades since I specialized in addiction medicine, and along with my team of nurses, I've guided countless detoxes for my patients. Our team noticed wide variability in patients' discomfort levels, when coming off narcotics, alcohol or sedatives. Sometimes the poor folks go through agony. Their expressions convey the most unbearable physical and psychological discomfort you can imagine. These unfortunates are cornered, restless, and exude hopelessness.

At the other end of the detox "feelz" spectrum, others breeze right through with only the slightest symptoms. They typically have a bright, positive mood, and complete their detox way ahead of schedule. At first, I thought this disparity was drug-type or habit-duration related. Years of a tough substance like heroin or Ambien would be hard for anyone to come off, right? But the drug didn't seem to matter.

I've watched heroin and methadone addicts with decades of a chronic habit, turn the page on a substance use in a few weeks—some in several *days*. I've witnessed patients drop a twenty-year alcohol habit it in a weekend. A little nervous, a bit sweaty, but cheerful the whole way. Still others never seem to figure it out, they abort a detox even when the worst of it is behind them. Why such a big difference? I think I know at least part of the reason: *philosophy*. Or said another way: what you think about how the world works, and your place in it. There's that word again, how does it apply to detox? Allow me to explain.

If your current detox is the *last* time you'll go ever go through withdrawal symptoms from stopping your substance habit, it will be surprisingly easy on you. If this is a temporary phase of abstinence, if you're headed soon back to managing your feelings with chemicals, then detox will be hell. *Why* you're bothering to go through the unpleasant symptoms affects *how* you experience withdrawal. It's not too different from most situations in life. If you've imagined that you'll do well in an upcoming challenge, say public speaking or an athletic competition, a positive mental picture helps you do better. If you're "psyched out," and worried you'll fail, then your performance will suffer. We live up—or down—to our own expectations.

But how does this account for different experiences of chemical withdrawal? *I thought that drugs were the cause of addiction,* you may be saying. I'm glad you asked. Our physical and emotional sensations are subjectively constructed. We have an internal "status monitor" of how we're doing, but meaning is shaped on the fly–as we experience the world. Our conclusions are strongly influenced by what our immediate perceptions are of danger or safety.

If you see a future without reliance on drugs to cope with life, if you imagine a bright, prosperous, happy horizon, then the physical discomfort and withdrawal symptoms are simply the price of admission to your new life. Detox is uncomfortable. Not going to sugar coat it; it sucks. And then bit by bit, gradually, it stops sucking.

But if you have no intention of fundamental change, if detox is your way to get the heat off and go through the motions, then each bit of physical discomfort is amplified. If you're spending a few days in Miserytown, with plans to return again soon, then your suffering is totally pointless. There is nothing worse than pointless suffering; it's the definition of torture.

I've also seen people veer between each mindset at different phases of their recovery. In the beginning, they may be well-motivated. Perhaps suffering a recent stinging humiliation which triggered an epiphany to finally quit for good. Not long after the newly clear-eyed soul gleans the slightest relief from the relentless treadmill of a substance habit, he begins negotiating. Bargaining with Nature or the detox nurse, our chap going through it wheedles for some relief. Perhaps, he thinks, he overreacted. His ego makes a full recovery .

He gets through the initial squeeze of quitting. He sees detox will work, and with enough time he'll get to zero. Once physical dependence is passed, the excuse to use again will be gone too. No more monkey on the back. Many detoxers reassess here. During a taper detox, when the psychological pinch starts to smart, they decide to stop weaning and instead try to maintain at a lower level. With a new insight that detox is *possible*, they paradoxically change their objective. Many times, soon after someone gets better, they recognize life will be different.

Once their friends and family know sobriety is possible for their loved one, they balk. They spit the bridle, and instead hope they can slink past claiming they have a disease outside of their personal control. Personal responsibility for your actions is the hallmark of passing from childhood to adulthood. So long as they continue to fail, the accountability bar seems, to them, much lower. If they stay sober, their family and friends will expect it in the future, remember.

I've also been humbled to watch people make a tentative start, but then build momentum as they go through detox. Building a "crew" of folks who support but do not judge is invaluable. Calling a friend who understands and simply listens to you moan and complain about how hard it is to grow up is frequently the lynchpin to a new life. This can happen simply reading stories of triumph and change too. Vicarious experience underpins Alcoholics Anonymous, and AA is chock-full of stories of those who've gone before you. Reading another's experience can give you a sense of context and direction and well as helping bolster your faith in the future. I hope some of the stories in this book have shown you how in so many ways we are all alike.

While we're praising Alcoholics Anonymous, they have an expression I like a lot: *life on life's terms*. We all must deal with challenges and unexpected hobbles on the road to our goals. The important thing is not in avoiding the impediment, the obstacle, but in moving toward it so you can grow. Ryan Holiday (and Marcus Aurelius) says the obstacle is the way. Don't wish life were easier, wish you were better, stronger, wiser, and more capable. When we show up for an opportunity to grow, change our understanding, to admit new ideas, we are alive often for the first time. Clearing away the old, dead wood, the ideas that no longer serve, is not just a practical matter, but is the journey of spirituality and meaning itself.

If your personal philosophy is that you have all you need in terms of understanding to be the best you can, then you are, as they say in Spanish, "tapado." In English, it translates to closed, sealed, the lid firmly in place. Maybe you'll agree, being *tapado* is the opposite of being humble. Humility is an awareness there is more to the situation than you perceive. Humble is teachable, allowing for new ideas and light to enter. The most important saying to come out of the Oracle at Delphi: Certainty, then Disaster. It's always wise to ask for guidance and perspective. We can't have others do our work for us, but we can seek their counsel and reduce the chance we'll make a mistake.

When life presents challenges, obstacles, and difficulties, we have an automatic, and evolutionarily ancient, categorization response. We auto-sort at a pre-conscious level, far below analytic understanding. A largely intact old brain (paleo brain) is in each of us. We evolved to do more complex tasks, and our neo-cortex (new brain) wraps around and relies the old one. Not only do we archive old habits in case we need them later, but the structure of the brain itself shows how precious any skill acquisition is. Face it, we're all hoarders of habits. You are quite animal-like, you run on instinct and survival programming, and you'll sacrifice the future to live today. I'm built the same way. Don't feel bad for being such an animal, we all are.

When we have the luxury of time and aren't under pressure, the neo-cortex (modern, higher brain) analyzes tricky problems and comes up with impressive solutions. The neo-cortex got us to the moon and did all your math homework. The paleo-cortex is where addiction resides. Its motives are more basic: survive and reproduce.

The three responses of the old-brain are *fight*, *flight*, or *freeze*. When challenged with something scary, one of our automatic responses is to fight back. In a pinch, this response can save your life. If you remember the story of the coyote and my little dog, you'll agree her fight response was triggered without a second thought. There is also the flight response, when something's terrifying and there are overwhelming odds, we flee. If the monsters are too big, running away is the smart move; live to fight another day.

The third option, often overlooked, is to freeze. Temporary paralysis turns the legs to stone; you don't want to make a wrong next move. You'll see animals do this right before they are pounced upon by a predator–they'll try to lie very still. The most extreme example may be the opossum, who famously "plays dead" to be less appetizing to its foe.

We play possum in our lives all the time, freezing and holding still, trying not to make matters worse. This is extremely common in relationships when they go down the same old path of argument and conflict. People know that they don't want to make things worse, but they don't know what to do next, so they freeze.

The ancient Greek myth of the medusa tells this tale well. Perseus, short a party gift, offered in a pinch to do anything for his host, Polydectes. The cunning rival spitefully sent young Perseus on a suicide mission: kill the un-killable gorgon. Although Medusa was mortal, she was said to be so hideous that looking directly at her headdress of snakes turned you instantly to stone.

Perseus was kitted out by his family, he was the son of Zeus after all. With a few bits of myth-tech (helm of invisibility, etc.), he dispatched Medusa and became king. He beheaded the poor gorgon and stuffed her head in a magic bag. Perseus was known to whip out the severed head to turn bad guys into stone if they got out of line.

I'm impressed with how relevant the Medusa parable is to our "freeze" response to fear. Medusa, remember, has her hair replaced with a nest of venomous snakes. Serpents, are symbols of chaotic danger and death. In *The Fruit, the Tree, and the Serpent: Why We See So Well,* primatologist Dr. Lynne Isbel of UC-Davis lays out the case that primate vision evolved most rapidly when venomous snakes lived with our primate ancestors up in the trees.

The time is around 60-80 million years ago. We evolved sharper vision to detect and deal with the only predator who could climb up to threaten us: serpents. We evolved an entire "snake detection circuit" made of enhanced color discrimination and pattern recognition, as well as movement detection. People, and primates, instinctively fear snakes without ever having seen them.

The Medusa story and Medusa-as-symbol have been used for everything from feminism to nihilism. In Jack London's book, *The Mutiny of the Elsinore*, in a prescient discussion of nihilism versus rational acceptance of individual responsibility, London observes:

> *"The profoundest instinct in man is to war against the truth; that is, against the real. He shuns facts from his infancy. His life is a perpetual evasion. Miracle, privilege of lifting the veil of Isis; men dare not. The animal, awake, has no fictional escape from the real because he has no imagination. Man, awake, is compelled to seek perpetual escape into hope, belief, fable, art, God, socialism, immortality, alcohol, love. From Medusa -- truth he makes an appeal to Maya -- lie."*

London's right; man will try to escape into anything he can to avoid confrontation with reality. Though I think complete reliance on rationalism, an atheistic approach, puts morality just out of reach, perpetual escape of any kind is the highway to dissipated oblivion. There is a higher manner of personal conduct to aspire toward. Striving daily toward it our lives not only have meaning, they're far more satisfying.

Believe it or not, at one point I was certain I wasn't going to survive much longer than about another two weeks. Maybe this wasn't an unreasonable conclusion to draw since I was injecting very powerful narcotics with regularity. I flirted with overdose a lot. I toyed with a very dangerous drug that could without warning leap up and (with apologies to Billy Collins) unman me with a snap. I didn't think I would be around to have to face the consequences of not facing the consequences. Believing I'd be dead soon, I made only short-term planning. My rolling actuarial estimate was so brief, I could let go of any responsibility for personal conduct. This is embarrassing to write two decades hence.

Of course, none of us knows when our allotted time is up, but impending-death as a personal philosophy preempts the need for accountability, truth telling, or growing up at all. If I don't plan, I can relive *Groundhog Day*, every day and make no progress.

Another pernicious personal philosophy is the extreme nihilism. I hear it said, "What difference will this make in a thousand years?" Imagine saying this to a child who suffered an injury? With a skinned knee, and a sobbing young kid, saying to her, "in a thousand years this won't make any difference, so stop crying." It's a futility mindset which disempowers us before we begin.

Who can say what the full effects of your actions today will be in one thousand years? Perhaps reading this book will cause you to think about your substance habits. Thinking may lead to permanent change, and then to a renewed love and closeness in your family. From there, support and self-sacrifice have fertile soil in which to bloom. Similarly, failure to turn your personal franchise around today may well portend the direst of consequences. The good news is you're responsible for your own life.

If we embrace the reductionist idea we are a meaningless speck on a meaningless rock in a meaningless universe, then no amount of personal accountability matters. We are doomed to drift pointlessly, and we might as well drink or kill ourselves, or each other for that matter.

I don't make here an admonition to adopt a specific religion, but without an inkling of higher power or order, it's much harder to chart a life of meaning. Personally, and as a man of science, I have doubts about an underlying order of the Universe. By the same token, when I contemplate something "under the rocks," as Norman Maclean called it, I feel better. Without taking a drug, simply considering an organizing principle for matter and energy makes me feel better. The cost: we should follow the rules or suffer the consequences.

Aesop's parable of the ant and the grasshopper, is worth touching on as we close this book. You'll remember that the ant and the grasshopper were work-friends, but they each had different philosophies. The grasshopper was very much a live-for-today kind of a fellow, enjoying the moment without a care for the future. As he comes upon his amigo lugging a giant ear of corn in the hot sun anthillward, he tries to convince the ant to come play with him in the grass.

The ant, fastidious as ever, sticks with his task and banks enough extra for the upcoming harsh season. The grasshopper plays all summer; he eats leaves until full, goofs off, and hangs out with friends. The grasshopper thinks "summer" all summer, while the ant thinks "winter" all summer. When the snows come, the ant holes up in its anthill, eats its stored food, and survives. The grasshopper, starving, not so much.

You have a philosophy, even if you don't think you do. Even though we may soak our minds in alcohol, drugs, work, or some new method of escape, we still ourselves in a certain light. And, even though we may pretend that there is no order in nature, we know, deep down, there must be. We each have a choice; let's choose to be all we can and give thanks to the mysterious Universe which gave us life.

I want to personally thank you for reading my book. No matter how many times I go through it, I always wish I could have said it better. But that's the way life is. I have two children, ages 19 & 17. As they're on the threshold of the world, I often feel like I need to cram in just one more story or explain to them another experience of how the world works. But they know what to do and so do you. Enough stories for now.

At a certain point, all parents must let go of their children. If you could get sober and change your habits purely on how much *I* want that for you, then everyone would be a success. But that's not how it works. I can only point toward the path, and I can only share my experience facing the dragon, but now I let go so you may slay your own beasts. I will tell you this: you're far more capable of change than you realize. Your habits were slowly built and must be slowly replaced.

If you'll allow me to say a prayer for you, I pray you'll stick with your own self-developed system for change. Take what you've learned in this book and amplify it with your own experience. Hang in there, even when though you'll have days when you feel like throwing in the towel. If your experience is like mine, in time you'll see your "mistakes" with a sense of humor and humility. We all have feet of clay.

And get out there and engage with the world. Trust at least one person and tell them the truth about your life and your experiences. Unburden yourself with the liberating gift of candor.

If I can answer any questions, field any complaints, or if you want to share your experience of habit change with me, feel free to drop me a line at: Jason@vhab.com

Until then remember, you're smarter than your addiction, and it doesn't want to kill you.

Find your mission and then help someone else find theirs.

All my best,

Jason Giles, MD

Malibu,   California.   September   2020.

Notes:

ABOUT THE AUTHOR

Dr. Giles grew up in Southern California. He studied Molecular Biology at UC Berkeley under his mentor Dr. Daniel Koshland.

He completed his medical degree and postdoctoral training in Sacramento at the UC Davis Medical center.

There he also met his wife, Rebecca when they were young doctors.

Dr. Giles returned to his hometown of Los Angeles to open his addiction medicine practice.

He considers himself blessed to have cheered many people in their quest to change substance habits.

Jason Giles is also the Founder and President of VHAB, Inc., the leading platform for behavioral health and habit change.

Dr. & Dr. Giles make their home in Los Angeles with their two children and three dogs.

www.ingramcontent.com/pod-product-compliance
Lightning Source LLC
Chambersburg PA
CBHW022334280326
41934CB00006B/634